Assessing
Educational Outcomes

Assessing Educational Outcomes

Third National Conference on Measurement and Evaluation in Nursing

Margery Garbin
Editor

National League for Nursing Press • New York
Pub. No. 15-2447

ISBN 0-88737-541-3

This book was set in Goudy by Publications Development Company. The editor and designer was Allan Graubard. Northeast Press was the printer and binder. The cover was designed by Lillian Welsh.

Printed in the United States of America

Contents

Contributors

Eunice A. Bell, PhD, RN, is Associate Professor of Nursing, Department of Graduate Nursing, Armstrong State College, Savannah, GA.

Anna Bersky, MS, RN, is CST Project Director, National Council of State Boards of Nursing, Chicago, IL.

Catherine A. Bevil, EdD, RN, is Associate Professor and Director, Baccalaureate Division, Department of Nursing, Thomas Jefferson University, Philadelphia, PA.

Janie Brown, EdD, RN, is Associate Professor, College of Nursing, Villanova University, Villanova, PA.

Betty J. Caffo, MS, RN, Chairperson, Department of Nursing, Wilmington College, New Castle, DE.

Sachiko Claus, PhD, RN, is Associate Professor, College of Nursing, Saginaw Valley State University, University Center, MI.

M. Louise Fitzpatrick, EdD, RN, FAAN, is Dean and Professor, College of Nursing, Villanova University, Villanova, PA.

Doris C. Ford, DSM, RN, is Associate Professor, Lurleen B. Wallace College of Nursing, Jacksonville State University, Jacksonville, AL.

Margery Garbin, PhD, RN, is Senior Vice President for Testing, National League for Nursing, New York.

Ann M. Gothler, PhD, MS, RN, is Professor of Nursing, Russell Sage College, Troy, New York.

Mary Graiver, MSN, RN, is Assistant Professor, College of Nursing, Saginaw Valley State University, University Center, MI.

Evelyn Dupree Guice, MSN, RN, is Assistant Professor, Lurleen B. Wallace College of Nursing, Jacksonville State University, Jacksonville, AL.

Mary Beth Hanner, PhD, RN, is Dean of Nursing Programs, Regents College, Albany, NY.

Novella Z. Keith, PhD, is Evaluation Consultant, Philadelphia, PA.

Linda Knecht, MSN, RN, is Assistant Professor of Nursing, Department of Nursing, University of Michigan, Flint, MI.

Sandra K. Krafft, EdD, RN, is Director, BSN Program, Hahnemann University, Philadelphia, PA.

Margaret Krawczyk, MSN, RN, is Assistant Professor, College of Nursing, Saginaw Valley State University, University Center, MI.

Carrie B. Lenburg, EdD, RN, FAAN, is President, Creative Learning and Assessment Systems.

Claire Manfredi, EdD, RN, is Associate Professor, College of Nursing, Villanova University, Villanova, PA.

Mary E. Periard, PhD, RN, is Assistant Professor of Nursing, Nursing Development and Research, Department of Nursing, University of Michigan, Flint, MI.

Theresa Valiga, EdD, RN, is Associate Professor and Director of the Graduate Program, College of Nursing, Villanova University, Villanova, PA.

Sr. Rachel Wallace, MSN, RN, is Associate Professor, College of Nursing, Saginaw Valley State University, University Center, MI.

Ellen A. Woodman, MS, RN, is Assistant Professor of Nursing and Director, Department of Nursing, University of Michigan, Flint, MI.

Mary M. Ziemer, DNSc, RN, is Associate Professor, College of Nursing, Villanova University, Villanova, PA.

Preface

The assessment movement within higher education grew rapidly during the past decade as a result of both internal and external pressures on academic improvement to better educate an increasingly diverse student population for an increasingly complex world. Externally, the public demanded reform and external accountability of institutions of higher learning.

A flurry of reports appeared during the mid-1980s concerning the state of higher education. These reports—by educational and governmental groups—had titles suggesting the need and urgency for change: *A Nation at Risk* (U.S. Department of Education, 1983), *To Reclaim a Legacy* (Bennett, 1984), and *Time for Results* (National Governors' Association, 1986), among others. The reports led to the implementation of outcomes assessment projects in several colleges and universities and by several state governments. By 1988, outcomes assessment was added to accreditation criteria by the Council on Postsecondary Accreditation and the U.S. Department of Education. With the recent addition of outcomes assessment to the National League for Nursing accreditation criteria, nursing joined the larger movement.

For outcomes assessment the unit of analysis is the program as a whole, rather than individual student outcomes. Nurse educators are accustomed to evaluating their overall program in regard to context (mission, objectives), input (resources), and process (procedures). Outcomes assessment of the program adds another dimension to the evaluation, measuring the extent to which the overall program purposes and objectives have been met.

In nursing education there is a strong tradition of assessing individual student outcomes. Mindful of the need to protect the public by assuring that graduates of the program possess the knowledge and abilities required for practice, nurse educators have become skilled in the use of teacher-made and standardized tests to evaluate knowledge, as well as clinical performance evaluation to examine actual task performance in naturalistic settings. Recently, nurse educators have moved toward the use of more qualitative approaches to measure affective outcomes of education and other complex phenomena, such as clinical judgment.

The move to outcomes assessment in nursing education requires a change of focus from evaluation of individual students to evaluation of the educational program as a whole. It means bringing faculty members together to identify the formative and summative evaluation processes already in place, then building on this base to develop a systematic process of collecting and analyzing data about program elements. Information gained through the evaluation process will ultimately be used to make decisions that will improve the quality and effectiveness of the program.

For any educational program, the process of developing a comprehensive outcomes evaluation program is imperfect. But in the very process of talking together, working through problems, and implementing an evaluation plan, important changes may occur. Hutchings (1987) gives the following advice:

> Do something even though it won't be perfect. Keep your eye on questions of validity and reliability but recognize, too, that it's in the process of working through admittedly imperfect plans for assessment that crucial changes may occur: outcomes are explicitly debated, questions about teaching get asked, faculty find new ways to think about their purposes, departments talk to each other, institutional identity grows stronger. . . . So do something, and whatever it is talk about it.

Faculty getting started on an assessment plan should keep in mind the long history of successful assessment practiced in nursing education. With this history and the resulting experience and expertise in the process of evaluation, nurse educators should emerge as natural leaders in the area of outcomes assessment in higher education.

Margery Garbin, PhD, RN

REFERENCES

Bennett, W. J. (1984). *To reclaim a legacy: A report on the humanities in higher education.* Washington, DC: National Endowment for the Humanities.

Hutchings, P. (1987). *Six stories: Implementing successful assessment.* Paper presented at the Second National Conference on Assessment in Higher Education. Washington, DC: American Association for Higher Education (reprint).

National Governors' Association. (1986). *Time for results: The governors' 1991 report on education.* Washington, DC: National Governors' Association.

U.S. Department of Education, National Commission on Excellence in Education. (1983). *A nation at risk: The imperative for educational reform.* (Report to the nation and the secretary of education). Washington, DC: U.S. Government Printing Office.

Introduction

In June 1991, the Third National Conference on Measurement and Evaluation in Nursing was sponsored by the National League for Nursing Test Service, prior to the NLN biennial convention in Nashville, Tennessee. The special focus on this conference—the assessment of educational outcomes—was selected in response to the questions and concerns expressed by nurse educators regarding the outcomes assessment of their programs. To meet the conference goals, papers were solicited in the following areas:

1. Theoretical and societal background of the movement to outcomes assessment in higher education.
2. Approaches to assessing the achievement of learning outcomes.
3. Directions for future development of assessment methodologies.

Two keynote speakers were invited to address the first area. For the other two areas, abstracts of relevant research were reviewed by select speakers. This effort resulted in a conference that addressed the most current issues and challenges of outcomes assessment.

The first two chapters provide a comprehensive overview of the topic. Novella Keith, a sociologist who gave the first keynote address (Chapter 1), "Assessing Educational Goals: The National Movement to Outcomes Evaluation," provides an historical overview, describing the external pressures as well as the internal changes in higher education leading to the current emphasis on assessment of learning outcomes. Dr. Keith discusses the relationship between assessment as measurement and assessment as "conversation" about teaching and learning, and how these two approaches to assessment are converging.

The second keynote speaker, Carrie Lenburg, in Chapter 2, "Assessing the Goals of Nursing Education: Issues and Approaches to Evaluation Outcomes," brings the focus directly to nursing education. Dr. Lenburg relates the link between key assessment concepts and the new NLN criteria for accreditation. She discusses the challenges faced by nurse educators in bringing about essential educational reform heralded by three current trends: the curriculum revolution focusing on caring; the assessment revolution emphasizing competence; and Nursing's Agenda for Health Care Reform, which emphasizes accountability. Dr. Lenburg's vision would integrate all three trends into a "cohesive and holistic system."

The next five papers present approaches to assessing learning outcomes. In Chapter 3, "Program Evaluation in Nursing Education: Creating a Meaningful Plan," Catherine Bevil describes the step-by-step process used by one nursing education program in developing and implementing a comprehensive program evaluation plan. Dr. Bevil describes a systematic approach built on an eclectic theoretical framework. She emphasizes the value of including stakeholders throughout the process, tailoring activities to existing structures, and capitalizing on existing human and material resources.

In Chapter 4, "An Outcome Assessment of Liberal Education for the Baccalaureate Nursing Major," Sachiko Claus *et al.* describe how one nursing education program participated in a university-wide outcomes project that was, in turn, part of a nation-wide project on outcomes assessment. In this research project, assessment instruments developed by the American College Testing Program were used to measure selected outcomes of a liberal education. The authors discuss the value and limitations of their research in the area of educational outcomes.

In Chapter 5, Ellen Woodman *et al.*, "Assessment of Affective Outcomes in RN/BSN Programs: Advancing Toward Professionalism," describe a research project to determine the relationship between selected personal, situational, and motivational factors and changes in professionalism that occur during the nursing education program. Variables in the affective domain, such as those reported here, are among the most important, albeit the most challenging to measure, outcomes of education in nursing.

In Chapter 6, "Validation Testing: Implications for RN-BSN Curriculum Development," Sandra Krafft and Betty Caffo discuss the performance of RN students on the NLN Mobility Profile II tests to validate prior learning for advanced placement in a baccalaureate nursing program. These tests measure nursing knowledge that RNs can be reasonably expected to have acquired through previous learning and experience. Drs. Krafft and Caffo discuss the implications of the finding that the RN students in their study performed better on the tests than the norms group of basic baccalaureate students.

Echoing a theme introduced by Carrie Lenburg in Chapter 2, Evelyn Guice and Doris Ford in Chapter 7 discuss "Developmental Programs and Remediation Strategies in Schools of Nursing." As students from diverse cultural and educational programs are increasingly recruited into nursing, the number of academically at-risk students also has increased. Successful completion of a program of study may depend on the availability of developmental and remediation programs to meet these students' needs. Guice and Ford describe the results of their survey of nursing programs to identify the kinds of strategies being used to assist at-risk students in one state.

The next two chapters suggest directions for future development of assessment methodologies. In Chapter 8, Anna Bersky describes "The Measurement Characteristics of Computerized Clinical Simulation Tests (CST)." The National Council of State Boards of Nursing is in the process of an extensive study of a CST model to measure clinical decision-making competence in nursing. The results of the CST pilot study described in Chapter 8 provide preliminary evidence that it is feasible to construct a valid and reliable CST examination of clinical decision-making ability. Depending on the results of further research on CST, it is quite possible that CST may be combined with computer adaptive testing (CAT) for nursing licensure examinations in the future.

In Chapter 9, another innovative measurement instrument is described by Ann Gothler and Mary Beth Hanner, "Development of an Instrument to Measure Thinking, Learning, and Creativity (TLC): A Triangulation Process." The instrument, consisting of five components, was designed to measure the effect of TLC on the perceived quality of work life and work satisfaction of registered nurses. The instrument was developed using triangulation—a multi-operation, multimethod approach in which quantitative and qualitative approaches are combined to more clearly understand the construct under study. The use of this methodology holds much promise for studying the complex phenomena of interest in nursing practice.

In the concluding Chapter 10, Mary Ziemer *et al.* report the results of a survey of "Curricula of Doctoral Programs in Nursing." In this study, the curriculum features defined as essential for a high quality doctoral program by the American Association of Colleges of Nursing were compared to the actual curricula of the doctoral programs surveyed. The authors discuss the implications of their findings in terms of the expected outcomes of doctoral education in nursing.

All these papers—from different approaches, perspectives, and settings—share a common purpose. They apply the principles of outcomes assessment to better assure that the graduates of nursing education programs will be the caring, competent, and accountable nurses intended by the program and needed by the public.

In closing, I extend a special thank you to all of the participants in the Third National Conference on Measurement and Evaluation in Nursing. Their excellent cooperation made possible the timely release of this publication. Special gratitude also is extended to Sally Barhydt, NLN's Assistant Vice President for Communications, and Allan Graubard, NLN's Senior Editor, for their expert assistance in preparing this book.

Margery Garbin, PhD, RN

1

Assessing Educational Goals: The National Movement to Outcomes Evaluation

Novella Z. Keith

In the mid-1980s, a new term entered the lexicon of higher education: *learning outcomes assessment.* To some, it was a tool with which to demonstrate and enhance the educational quality of institutions of higher learning. Clearly stated expectations for what students should learn and be able to do by the end of a program of studies ("learning outcomes"), coupled with sound information about the extent of their achievement ("assessment"), should serve well the cause of improving performance. To others, it represented one more bureaucratic intrusion, misguided and mindless at best, Machiavellian at worst, a requirement for testing that would erode the very ground on which excellence in higher education rested: a high degree of professionalism with its correspondingly high classroom autonomy, and the freedom of faculty and institutions to expose students to a rich diversity of materials and perspectives.

1

In the intervening years between then and now, the debate this new trend engendered has not ceased. Whether from proponents or detractors, assessment continues to evoke strong feelings. Several things have changed, however. For one, it has become increasingly evident that assessment ought not be considered merely a passing fad. One may cite as evidence the prevalence of assessment mandates or "recommendations" from state-level officials and professional organizations and the growing number of institutions with assessment initiatives (see Figure 1-1). One also may cite, as an indication of the potential for permanence, the context in which assessment has emerged—a context of crisis and transformation of our society, which assigns a potentially new and vital role to education. It seems to me, however, that the causes for the persistence of assessment go beyond these events, important though they are. Assessment has "staying power" because it raises a fundamental, enduring question that goes to the core of the educational enterprise: what are students actually learning in our schools.

This question is not only fundamental; it is, or ought to be, of profound interest to educators. Perhaps the early emphasis on external mandates—the way most educators became aware of assessment—initially prevented educators from seeing this. But now, after some seven years of exploration and practice, our understanding of assessment and its uses has expanded. Outcomes assessment is not especially about administering tests, primarily to demonstrate learning and thus be accountable to one's constituencies. Nor is it merely "any process of gathering concrete evidence about the impact and functioning of undergraduate education" (Boyer and Ewell, n.d.). These aspects of assessment exist, but miss a vital ingredient that injects life into the process: assessment is a "conversation about teaching and learning." The assessment discourse has altered significantly, as a shift has occurred from emphasis on precise and systematic *measurement* to emphasis on the *uses* of assessment to improve learning. Thus the assessment questions, "what are students learning" and "how do we know," have led us down a path that reasserts the centrality of the teaching mission of higher education, insisting that teaching and learning must matter.

These two themes—the shifting assessment discourse and the rekindling of the teaching mission—form the core of this study. Surveying assessment from such vantage points should help shape what should be a positive, even enthusiastic, response to the mandate that now faces all educators. We will doubtless encounter difficulties along the way as in any other change-oriented endeavor. We also will find that, if we link outcomes assessment firmly to teaching as a value, if we integrate it into ongoing departmental activities and faculty discussions, outcomes assessment can make an important contribution to enhancing students' learning.

ASSESSMENT'S "STAYING POWER": THE SHIFTING DISCOURSE

It has become commonplace to cite economic, demographic, and other pervasive societal pressures impinging directly or indirectly on higher education as
the underlying "causes" of assessment. It is then assumed that, because these
trends are enduring, the movement they generated also must be lasting. Yet
this logic does not necessarily follow. My approach, instead, will be to review
these societal trends to trace the shifting definitions of assessment to the
discovery of its connectedness to our fundamental questions and values.

American society has been undergoing vast changes since the 1970s, the
impact of which will be felt well into the next century. The main manifesta-
tions of these changes are familiar to most educators: increasing pressures on
the economy as we advance into an era of global competition; maintenance of
American global dominance through military over specifically economic
means; technology outstripping our ability to understand and control it; increasing numbers of children living in poverty, especially among people of
color; demographic shifts, such as the growing age of the population and the
growing presence of current "minorities" who are expected to comprise some
40 percent of the American population by the year 2050 (Kellogg, 1988).

These changes and their ripple effects are touching all social institutions.
Political alignments, the role of all levels of government, the social class structure, the organization of business entities, health care, and, yes, education are all
feeling the pressure and experiencing or anticipating vast transformations.[1]
When seen as a whole, these changes speak of the end of an era: American
society has to be reconstructed. Old formulas no longer seem to work and,
while new ones are beginning to emerge, in the process there is much confusion
and uncertainty. Assessment emerges as a potentially new construct growing
out of the tensions of the old system.

External Pressures Toward Assessment

The 1970s were indeed a turning point for the American economy. The
technological lead eroded, growth effectively halted, foreign competition increased, a much larger rate of unemployment prevailed than had been considered acceptable in the post-war period, and real incomes and standards of
living declined.[2] The new stage in the international division of labor coun-
selled economic restructuring based on information and communications,

high technology, and service industries. As the governor of Arkansas put it, the American economy had lost its competitive advantage in three of four areas: productivity, a vast and captive home market, and natural resources. The only advantage left, according to the governor, was "a core of really bright people and a core of institutions of higher education that are creating new things for people to do all the time" (Clinton, 1988, p. 4). Other governors joined the chorus: "if America is to succeed as a nation, education will be the linchpin to it all . . . . It's going to take brainpower for us to compete in world markets" (Marchese, 1988). The educational establishment was called upon to play a dual role in easing the transition: provide a workforce with the requisite knowledge and skills—to help the United States "become a nation of people who think for a living" (Tucker, cited in Edgerton, 1987, p. 4)—and contribute to economic development, largely through its research and knowledge-generating functions (see, for instance, Groennings, 1987, on New England). The policy question, of course, was how to achieve such results.

Two related factors in the immediate environment provided the context in which the new roles of higher education would be forged. First, budgetary pressures at the federal level caused the shifting of responsibility for many social programs onto state and local governments, the largesse of corporations, private charities, and the American public. This was at the same time that, for many of the above, the economic and fiscal crisis created pressures of its own.[3] Second, the new, heightened expectations of the educational system would have to be met largely through reallocation—and in intense competition with other social needs—rather than through growing resources, as had been the pattern from the 1950s to the early 1970s—the "golden age" of American higher education (Keller, 1983, p. 8).

The capacity of the research universities to generate knowledge was well established and simply needed to be selectively supported. Business-higher education partnerships and the entrepreneurial propensities of faculty would augment public efforts. Improving student learning was a much more difficult policy question. Here, a new climate of closer public scrutiny of undergraduate education was emerging—scrutiny from consumers paying a greater share of costs, from legislators faced with difficult choices about program funding, from the business world, to which development officers were increasingly turning, and, last but not least, from academic leaders.

Earlier, accountability to external audiences—accrediting bodies, oversight agencies, and the public at large—had been defined largely in terms of input measures: maintaining adequate resources such as libraries and laboratories, employing appropriately trained faculty, and using sound fiscal management practices. Professional accrediting bodies, such as the National League for Nursing, also stipulated certain requirements concerning the curriculum. By the 1980s, however, definitions of effectiveness and efficiency in higher education were changing. The careful husbanding of resources and timely accumulation of credits were no longer deemed sufficient evidence that learning had taken place. Statements of intent about the knowledge and experiences to which students would be *exposed* had to give way to assumption of responsibility about what the students would actually *learn*.[4]

In the meantime, however, for the purposes of the "new" accountability, assessment was a way to give greater emphasis to student performance as a measure of institutional effectiveness, and new demands on institutions to demonstrate their students' achievements in public ways. For public institutions, this has taken mainly the form of assessment mandates or "recommendations" from state-level officials—as Mingle (1989) has noted, an attempt by states to achieve academic quality through nontraditional regulation rather than by "buying it." This was one thread in the yet-to-be woven fabric of outcomes assessment.

Whether because of institutional priorities, the demonstration effect of public mandates, later mandates from accrediting and professional organizations, or other causes, many private colleges and universities also have initiated outcomes assessment. Although the movement has been swift—by 1990, 82 percent of institutions of higher learning stated they were involved in some form of assessment—what is covered by the term varies greatly. Figure 1–1 provides a chronology of major assessments "events."

1972	Alverno College—"assessment of learning."
1973	Northeast Missouri State College (later University)—"value added" assessment.
1984	Florida—state mandated "gatekeeping" assessment ("sophomore test").
1985	Tennessee introduces "incentive funding."
1985	First annual Conference on Assessment in Higher Education.
1985	AAHE Assessment Forum is formed.
1986	Southern Regional Education Board—starts trend of outcomes assessment in accreditation.
1987	Virginia mandates campus-based assessment; New Jersey assessment mandates through College Outcomes Evaluation Program, including sophomore-level state-mandated assessment instruments; almost one-fourth of states promoting or requiring outcomes assessment at undergraduate level.
1987, 1988	Outcomes assessment added to accreditation criteria by Council on Postsecondary Accreditation and U.S. Department of Education.
1990	Four-fifths of states promoting assessment, majority following Virginia model; 82 percent of institutions reporting assessment underway.

Figure 1–1
Chronology of Higher Education Assessment "Events"

Much of the assessment discourse in the legislative arena was, as we have seen, strongly utilitarian in ways that rankle the academic vision. Surely, economic development and job preparation should not be the principal yard-sticks with which our efforts are measured! Figure 1-1 alludes to the existence of alternative visions for assessment, some of which already had a considerable history of their own. Yet we should not discount the importance of the utilitarian probings. In posing the question, even if in a limited framework, external audiences created the necessity—the professional responsibility—for a concerted inquiry into "higher" learning: if not this, then what?

State assessment mandates, some of which were developed with the partici-pation of the academic community, vary considerably in their approach to "knowing how much students learn" and "improving student learning." Among the early mandates, the "Virginia model" confines itself to requiring institutions to undertake assessment, stating explicitly that the purpose is to improve student learning rather than compare colleges. The mandate provides some guidelines—for instance, campuses should pay attention to general edu-cation, remediation, the major, alumni follow-up, and should provide evi-dence of "results" (i.e., strengthening areas of weakness, etc.)—but leaves the identification of appropriate learning goals and decisions on implementation to each institution. Quite a different spirit characterizes Florida's initiative. Following the pattern of the K-12 system, the state requires administration of a series of standardized tests to all sophomores in public higher education or receiving state financial aid. This has been called a gatekeeping test because students failing to achieve preestablished scores are eventually prevented from continuing with junior-level studies. New Jersey has combined a more direc-tive "Virginia model" for campus-based assessment with a state-mandated sophomore assessment of "general intellectual skills" (GIS), to be used for evaluation and improvements in institutions rather than for gatekeeping.[5] Finally, Tennessee provides fiscal incentives to institutions that, first, imple-ment a program of student testing, and, over time, show improvements in student scores.

The mandates generally include improving college-level student learning as a major objective, but in so doing also reveal implicit or explicit visions of the crucial content of that learning and the locus of responsibility for ensuring improvements. Note that the locus of responsibility is important not only from a political perspective but also because the needs of the decision-makers shape the type of assessment data to be collected. The message of Florida's CLAST, a state-level test of basic language and math skills, is the whittling away of faculty authority and a reductionism of the college curriculum. In emphasizing scores on a few tests, selected, however, by institutions and faculty, Tennessee also evinces a rather simplistic view of student learning. New Jersey's GIS, an ensemble of some ten short-answer-type instruments, constitutes a much more sophisticated and comprehensive view of the first two-years of college-level learning. However, assessment data are not reported in ways that facilitate the making of meaningful connections to the curriculum. The control exercised by the state on the assessment makes improving student learning a matter of central policy moreso than faculty discussion.

To the relief of most academicians, the vast majority of assessment mandates, by both states and professional associations (including the National League for Nursing) has followed the general outlines of the rather benevolent and unobtrusive approach of the state of Virginia. According to the latest survey of state initiatives (Ewell, Finney, & Lenth, 1990, p. 5), "the overwhelming public posture for state assessment remains 'improvement,' not 'accountability.'" Generally, this leaves both the content of student learning and the implementation of improvements to the colleges themselves. We should bear in mind, however, that since assessment is the tool of a "new" accountability, the state leaders' distinction between *improvements* and *accountability* may be little more than an exercise in semantics.

The road travelled to this point, in the face of competing paths that either prescribe a view of learning or preempt an important faculty role, may offer a map-in-the-making for policy development in an uncertain, new environment. It is punctuated with discussion, sometimes acrimonious but always revealing, about what students should learn and the "levers of change" available to people located at different levels of the system to try to improve that learning.

So far, the major contribution from outside the academy has come in the form of asking relevant questions to spark the discussion and insisting on a bona fide search for answers. Significant segments of the academic community have responded, entering early into the dialogue (through such activities as the Assessment Forum of the American Association of Higher Education). At their best, they are making the questions their own and are thus steering the movement in directions responsive to outside demands but also congruent with sound educational precepts. And, so far, state leaders have generally demonstrated a willingness to listen and change tracks when necessary.

I stated earlier that external mandates were only one thread in the fabric of assessment. To broaden the picture, we need, first, to look at other factors that sparked questioning and self-reflection within the academy and the higher education community, and, second, to place the development of "solutions" in a dynamic context, one in which we can see the process not as an imposition but as a convergence—an appropriation, even—of the meaning of educational quality.

Changes in the Academy: Assessment as an
Internal Response

I have already noted the vast expansion of higher education between 1955 and 1974. This period witnessed not only a 350 percent increase in the number of students in college, but also, as is well known, a vast increase in diversity— diversity of institutions (witness the birth of community colleges), of students, and of curricula (black studies, women studies, and so on). By the early 1970s, however, there was growing concern, as other sources of malaise were added to the emerging economic problems.

Demographic trends and the competition for students. Demographics were at the origins of one problem. It was not difficult, after all, to peruse the figures on births and note that there would be one-fourth fewer 18-year-olds by the mid-1990s than there were in the late 1970s. In the context of already pressing financial difficulties, experts predicted a decline of 10 to 30 percent in the number of institutions by the later date—this would translate into the closing or merger of some 300 to 900 institutions.[6]

As we now know, these dire predictions have not come to pass. Enrollments actually increased—though not at earlier rates—from 9,757,000 undergraduates in 1978 to 11,304,000 in 1988. Most private colleges, even the small and struggling ones, have managed to survive and even prosper. Strong recruitment programs and special efforts to respond to student needs have figured prominently among the factors accounting for the relative success. Most of all, however, according to O'Keefe (1989, p. 19), credit must be given to those institutional leaders who heeded "warnings about potential enrollment declines, identified particular needs and opportunities, . . . and *did* something about it." In other words, proactive institutional leadership can and will make a crucial difference—perhaps there is something to the old adage about viewing crises as challenges rather than problems.

Manifold initiatives were introduced to manage the anticipated crisis: retention programs, special services for a growing adult student population, aggressive recruitment, inventive use of facilities, and, yes, assessment. To what purposes? The times called forth two very different constructs of assessment: as feedback to improve learning and as student performance data to demonstrate the worth of an institution. It is instructive, in this regard, to review the experiences of Alverno College (Milwaukee) and Northeast Missouri State University, two assessment pioneers.

Not unlike many of the early external mandates, Northeast Missouri State University construed assessment as a "report card," one that hopefully would earn it rewards in the form of improved reputation and greater resources. Starting in 1972, NMSU began developing an alternative approach to demonstrating excellence: "value added." This approach focuses on student learning gains between entering and leaving an institution, as measured by standardized examinations.[7] Students were required to take tests such as the ACT Freshman College Entrance Exam and, as seniors, the ETS Graduate Records Exam in their major. Aggregated test results were then used for departmental and institutional planning rather than for specific, instructionally-oriented feedback to individual students and their teachers. In particular, such data could demonstrate the relative standing of one's graduates compared to those of similar institutions. Assessment data were used, in fact, to raise the institution's standing, and figured in the successful change of Northeast Missouri's mission from a teachers college to a comprehensive university.

Although Northeast Missouri achieved its goals, this type of assessment raises several questions. Giving prominence to results (the "report card") may lead to assessment "driving" the curriculum, yet it is not here that the fundamental problem lies. All assessment tends to shape what students actually learn, which is why good teachers make sure they assess all important aspects of learning. In an interesting book that focuses on assessment as a way of *knowing* students, Rowntree (1987) proposes that the ways an educational system assesses its students say a great deal about what it values and the extent to which it strives to accomplish what it professes.[8] A national test may measure some important facets of learning but hardly all. It is the overemphasis on ensuring success on any partial measure—as with the Florida or Tennessee mandates—that is the source of the problem. Our colleagues from the K-12 system know this all too well. Encouraged by the growing assessment discourse, NMSU has since broadened its own approach to assessment.

Beyond the partial nature of the test, there is the problem of comparison. On the one hand, comparison is essential to getting a sense of where one stands. Completing a doctorate in three years is tantamount to doing it with lightning speed, only because most people take "forever." On the other hand, some kinds of comparisons can create mischief—as when adolescents tell their parents that "*everybody's* room is messy and you should see so and so's!" The retort should be, of course, that there are standards, after all, that are not affected by what "everybody is doing." The first type of comparison is "norm-referenced"; the second is "criterion-referenced." Norm-referenced assessments invite comparison through competition with others—and competition does not necessarily ensure excellence, ideology notwithstanding. Although the data may be analyzed in other ways, their chief contribution is to produce a *ranking* of test takers, complete with winners and losers (49 percent must be below average). As is true of our typical grading system, all other information about learning is lost. Criterion-based comparisons, on the other hand, measure one's performance with regard to established criteria without concern, in theory, for what the average accomplishment might be. They provide a richer source of information regarding what students are and are not learning. Criterion-referenced assessment also can help students evaluate their own achievement and have a clear sense of what they need to learn in order to improve their performance. Perhaps much of the early discourse about assessment was concerned about "ranking" because, after all, a "report card" mentality is the most pervasive legacy of our educational system.

Unlike Northeast Missouri, Alverno College placed Rowntree's injunction at the heart of its assessment program. In 1972, Alverno was one of the "small and struggling" private colleges faced with the necessity to define and demonstrate their worth—or face decline. Discussions undertaken then, to explore "the meaning and purpose of liberal education at Alverno," were shaped by the question, "what are the outcomes [of education] for the student, rather than the input by the faculty?" (Alverno College, 1987, p. 3) The result was an innovative curriculum structured by eight competence areas ("abilities"), each with six sequenced levels of development, and featuring a combination of course-based and out-of-course assessments for each competence level.

While Alverno was unique in many ways—its abilities included critical thinking, global responsibility, and effective citizenship long before these became fashionable in higher education circles—two characteristics of its assessment program make it especially noteworthy. The first is the college's insistence on assessment as primarily an adjunct to the learning of individual students—and only secondarily as a means to demonstrate the worth of curricula, programs, and the institution as a whole. Rather than a report-card mentality we have a mentoring mentality. The second is the early understanding that an integrated curriculum requires the occasional use of assessments that are not course-based but offer the students and the faculty an opportunity for a more encompassing understanding of what students are learning.

Alverno showed the possibilities inherent in a shift in assessment practices at all levels. Today, the college is flourishing and its graduates are well-respected in the local community. Its approach, while not fully replicated anywhere, continues to inform the national discourse about assessment, constantly reasserting its integral link with teaching and learning.

Of new curricula and student learning. The second source of malaise in higher education had to do with the curriculum, not only in the usual sense of what was taught, but also in the sense of what was learned. The growth and changes of the 1960s had left a legacy of curricular fragmentation and overspecialization. Starting with *A Nation at Risk* in 1983, the 1980s were a decade of intense scrutiny and activity, as a spate of national reports on the state of higher education was matched by intense activity on campuses. A list of the major national reports and selected reports on professional programs is reproduced in Figure 1–2.

YEAR	REPORT	SPONSOR/AUTHOR
1983	A Nation at Risk	U.S. Dept. of Education
1984	Physicians for the 21st Century	Association of American Colleges
1984	Involvement in Learning	National Institute of Education
1984	To Reclaim a Legacy	National Endowment for the Humanities (Bennett Report)
1985	Integrity of the College Curriculum	American Association of Colleges
1985	Higher Education and the American Resurgence	Carnegie Foundation for the Advancement of Teaching (Newman Report)
1985	American Business Schools: Priorities for Change	Business-Higher Education Forum
1986	A New Vitality in General Education	American Association of Colleges (Joseph Katz, chair)
1986	Time for Results	National Governors Task Force on College Quality
1986	A Nation Prepared: Teachers for the 21st Century	Carnegie Forum on Education and the Economy

Figure 1-2
Major Reports of 1980s

While the focus of each report is different, there are remarkable areas of agreement. The response to the crisis of the late twentieth century has been a serious discussion about the role of higher education and, in particular, a rethinking of the aims for student learning in anticipation of future needs. Without diminishing the importance of in-depth knowledge, as acquired through a major area of study, there is a strong emphasis on enabling students to integrate what they know and put it in a broad perspective. The focus is not only on given knowledge, but on the processes and methods through which it is acquired. This has been taken to mean that the *whole* curriculum should be designed to develop in students certain intellectual capacities—critical thinking, problem solving, independent learning, ethical reasoning—and personal qualities (for instance, creativity, openness to change, adaptability, tolerance for diversity, civic mindedness).

One thing that distinguishes these efforts from earlier periods of academic soul searching has been the echoing, within the academy, of the new concern about "results" from outside its walls. For instance, after discussing the decline and devaluation of college degrees,[9] faculty responsibilities, and the curriculum, *Integrity in the College Curriculum* addresses outcomes assessment in a section entitled "The Problem of Accountability," (American Association of Colleges, 1985, p. 33):

One of the most remarkable and scandalous aspects of American higher education is the absence of traditions, practices, and methods of institutional and social accountability . . . . How can colleges and universities assure the American people and themselves that they are doing what they say they are doing? How does anyone know that the curriculum really "works"? There must be ways of demonstrating to state legislatures, students, and the public at large that the colleges know what they are doing (or do not know) and that they are doing it well (or poorly). The colleges themselves must be held responsible for developing evaluations that the public can respect.

There are three main areas of assessment . . . : students, programs, faculty. In all three, interrelated as they are and by necessity requiring concurrent attention, the professors are fundamentally responsible and therefore charged with designing and monitoring the mechanisms of assessment [my emphases].

Such themes are repeated, with variations, in most of the other reports. Their message is uniform. Higher education is poised on the edge of a crisis of public confidence and should take the call to accountability seriously. This means accepting assessment in the spirit of professional self-evaluation and self-regulation. There is a basis, here, for dialogue with assessment proponents from outside the academy, but the assessment question has not been fully appropriated. It is rather like agreeing to take the medicine oneself rather than having it forced down one's throat.

In speaking only in terms of accountability, the report of the American Association of Colleges (1985) missed an important connection between the new curricular emphases and the assessment movement—a connection that was not only logical but would align assessment with something of value to academicians: the curriculum. If the curriculum is seen as a whole, with a premium on the students' ability to integrate knowledge from many different sources and make it their own, and if one questions the wisdom of degrees based on the accumulation of credits, then it should follow that new forms of evaluating student learning are needed, practices that focus, for instance, on cumulative, integrated knowledge, such as may be attained as a result of several courses, course clusters, or an entire program of study. This was, indeed, one of Alverno's conclusions. Course-level examinations may meet these criteria, of course, but are most likely to do so only in clearly sequenced programs of study, as in many of the professions and sciences. Curriculum revisions may produce no more than wishful thinking unless they are matched by assessments that answer the simple question: are students learning what we think we are teaching them? In this sense, assessment belongs equally to institutions that need to "make a case" for themselves and to the most prestigious ones. Derek Bok (1986), president of Harvard, makes this point in his book *Higher Learning*:

> . . . *efforts to improve our colleges have produced only modest results in helping students progress toward the academic goals of a liberal education . . . . [These] findings are not terribly surprising . . . . The fact remains that the time faculties and administrators spend working together on education is devoted almost entirely to considering what their students should study rather than how they can learn more effectively or whether they are learning as much as they should. The professors who vote for new majors or curricular reforms know very little about whether these initiatives will actually help students progress toward the educational goals of the institution. And rarely, if ever, do they make a serious effort to find out.* (pp. 57–58)

Assessment is thus set squarely at the center of academic life. Its purpose?—to serve educational and pedagogical endeavors; to demonstrate the contributions of a liberal education, and thus broaden the earlier, utilitarian vision. There are, of course, many ways to accomplish this goal. The importance of this major shift in purpose is not that it ends the discussion but that it changes the face of assessment, substantially shedding its bureaucratic look and revealing its potential as a valuable adjunct to our primary task.

Does this mean that accountability is no longer an issue? The answer is no. The need to assure external audiences about student learning, to reassert the value of college degrees, remains. As the ex-governor of New Jersey, Thomas Kean (an "education governor"), put it in an address to the New Jersey higher education community, entitled "Time to Deliver,"

> *You have promised . . . that your graduates will have the knowledge and abilities to be productive in their work —a prerequisite not only of national strength but individual fulfillment.*
>
> *Maybe you never said those promises aloud. But we heard them nevertheless . . . .*
>
> *[Your critics] say that higher education promises much and delivers too little . . . . The public wants you to prove the critics wrong: You can.* [10]

There is, then, an unspoken compact. For the time being, at least, accountability can be satisfied by foregoing the "report card" approach and reporting, instead, on the steps taken toward improvements, in ways that convey that the task is undertaken earnestly and in the spirit of professionalism.

What Have We Learned?

The shift witnessed in the last seven years can be described as a movement from accountability to improvements (or summative vs. formative evaluation) but also from concern with measurement to concern with use. The two poles are not necessarily mutually exclusive, but a tendency toward one or the other will call forth different assessment tasks and challenges. At the risk of over-simplification, let me bifurcate the concept:

1. *Assessment as measurement*: the principal focus is on the *technical* task of designing psychometrically sound instruments, primarily for the purpose of producing a "report card," whose purpose is to rank and sort. Technical expertise is needed.

2. *Assessment as "conversation"*: here the principal focus is on enhancing learning, whether by focusing on the individual student as learner or on the aggregate effects of a curriculum or program of study. This focus recognizes the complexity of the web connecting measurement and improvements and the crucial role that collegial inquiry must play in the process of discovery and "solution." This approach puts a premium on the organizational and human relations skills that involve people in a conversation about teaching and learning and promotes shared responsibility for student learning.

The movement toward the second focus has produced many models. Of course, from the beginning there was the model set by Alverno, in which assessment is so integral to each student's educational process that it becomes itself a tool for teaching and learning.[11] There is the "classroom assessment" model developed by Pat Cross and Thomas Angelo, of interest to individual faculty, since they can use assessment in their courses to help them obtain immediate feedback on what their students are and are not learning—and sharing their findings with the students.[12] There is assessment designed to bridge the gap between what is taught and what is learned at the academic program level—that is, assessment for the formative evaluation and improvement of the curriculum.[13]

One or two years ago, I would have said that the last was the model of choice for most faculty. Now, the lines of demarcation between models are becoming increasingly blurred, as assessment practitioners raise new questions and explore the potential for integrating all of their activities as teachers.[14] Professional programs, for instance, offer particularly good opportunities for combining individual student assessment (for instance, evaluation of performance in practice settings) with assessment of the program's learning outcomes, since there tends to be more agreement among faculty on the contents and learning goals of at least some program courses.[15] One thing is certain: the fluidity of approaches and ongoing experimentation are a constant invitation to explore and expand assessment's potential contribution.

At this point, we need to insert some sobering facts. The "second option" of assessment has stimulated much interesting discussion and creative activity. More than a fait accompli, however, it represents a possibility, an opportunity that many have seized to work toward significant change in the academy. It has not been universally embraced. Involvement in assessment has been growing and involvement does seem to increase positive views toward assessment.[16] Some 50 percent of respondents to an annual survey by the American Council on Education (*Campus Trends*, 1990) believe that assessment "will significantly improve undergraduate education" and there is a palpable feeling of excitement among the growing numbers who attend national assessment conferences. Still, 73 percent of respondents to the same ACE survey continue to fear misuse. And, according to an estimate by Peter Ewell, probably the most knowledgeable (and certainly the most widely travelled) national expert, in the states that have assessment mandates, around 15 percent of campuses are making good progress, another 15 percent are "totally at sea," and the rest are "complying as best [they] can" (cited in Hutchings & Marchese, 1991, p. 34).

There is a sort of summing up that comes easily when one has participated in the assessment movement since its dawning and has heard the conversation— and the heckling—from all sides. It comes out of the depths, in the form of comments one might have heard (all references to any living or working persons are purely fictitious). "Can we compile an institutional report card? What about national educational indicators?" asked an unnamed government official of his measurement expert. "Why do we have to do this?" said the president to the official, the chairman to the dean, the professor to the chairman, and the student to the professor. "If you insist that we do it, tell us how. Are there any tests we can use?" retorted some professors and perhaps some presidents (while the others just looked away). "Wait, wait, there is something to this," said a couple of strangers from places no one had ever heard of. Others joined in: "let's give it a try . . ." And so they started talking, and experimenting. "A bunch of happy amateurs," commented a friendly social scientist, "but they're onto something." Said the government officials, "well, as long as they're working to improve, it's fine with us. But if not . . . ." (some still secretly wished for their indicators, but they couldn't say it aloud). And, as the happy "amateurs" worked, they eliminated or solved some problems.

In fact, these "amateurs" determined that, in order to link assessment and improvements, assessment must:

- Answer questions people care about.
- Be owned by the faculty.
- Be specifically linked to the curriculum and the classroom.

- Be a means to an end and not an end in itself.
- Involve collaboration.
- Occur in a context that facilitates change: the culture of an institution or department, its values and system of rewards—all these are paramount.

And, as the happy "amateurs" worked, they also discovered new challenges.

NEW ISSUES FOR ASSESSMENT

The availability of a good thermometer does not produce health. Health is the product of a supportive environment. While shifting the discourse toward the fundamental and enduring questions raised by the second approach helps insert assessment at the center of the academic enterprise, success also creates new problems. Having started out trying to find or develop a few good instruments, one finds oneself with the vastly more complex undertaking of fostering a community that is truly supportive of teaching and learning. In many academic settings, this is tantamount to tackling academic culture change. We have exchanged a technical task, that could have been assigned to the measurement experts, for an organizational one that we can only do ourselves. Figure 1–3 provides an introduction to the new task, offering some insights (a thorough discussion would be impossible in this context) that might be of help when venturing into assessment.[17]

Departments and campuses vary greatly. Some institutions are heavily bureaucratic, others are more collegial. One's department colleagues may collaborate easily and frequently, while another department may be like many a family, whose members get along because they know how to avoid the issues that cause conflict. These differences notwithstanding, we can speak of an academic culture, with dominant tendencies, values, norms, and the like. Its standard bearer remains the research university and its most valued activity is scholarly writing . . . of the kind that gives rise to many publications. Teaching, which is generally valued by faculty (Austin & Gamson, 1983), is very much an individual activity and pedagogy and its kindred interests do not usually appear on the agenda of department meetings or as items of discussion at faculty lunches.

When we compare these cultural tenets to the cultural requirements of "assessment as conversation," it becomes obvious that the latter constitute a significant departure. Yet, if the new task is to succeed, it must evoke a modicum of collaboration, of sharing, and opening one's classroom doors.

ACADEMIC CULTURE	ASSESSMENT REQUIREMENTS
Individualistic: the department is best that coordinates least	*Coordinated* efforts
Solitary work	*Collaborative*
Rewards *research* and *publication* over teaching	Much effort to be expended on activities related to *teaching*
Values *teaching* (even in research universities)	Values *teaching* and *learning*
Oriented to passing on the *discipline* and disciplinary knowledge (latent goal: recreating the professor)	Oriented toward *learning outcomes*—whether students have obtained needed skills and knowledge
Boundaries of own classroom are *closely guarded*	Faculty agree to include in own courses themes, issues, assessments of interest to department and share course information as needed
Self-monitoring (peer professionals and self)	*Self*-monitoring and *accountability*
Great variety of activities and demands: produces intrinsic satisfaction but also role strain	*Time* (especially in early stages)

Figure 1-3
Characteristics of Academic Culture and
Assessment Requirements

And it must be nurtured by a culture that truly values and rewards it. How can we begin to close the gap? Here are some thoughts and approaches for your consideration.

First, cultures are not monolithic. The assessment "movement" has, in fact, joined a growing "subcultural" chorus whose themes are learning communities, collaborative learning, mentoring, the "scholarship of teaching"—whose agenda is to reassert the centrality of teaching and learning in all of higher education.[18] Even discipline-based associations, traditionally the bastions of research-based definitions of excellence, have begun to focus in greater numbers on teaching and undergraduate education.

This leads me to a second point. Change certainly needs to occur at the level of the system as a whole—for instance, by attaching significant rewards to good teaching and eliminating the perils frequently associated with a preference for teaching. However, the need for systemic change should not prevent educators from initiating changes in our own environment (i.e., department or institution). If the assessment movement offers any lesson in this regard, it is that we have the ability to influence the course of events, especially when relatively new initiatives, such as assessment, are as yet somewhat unformed and would-be participants—from governors, to accrediting agencies, to provosts and faculty—are still groping to find models for implementation.

There remains, of course, the matter of change within the department. "Assessment as conversation" requires collaboration, a willingness to give up some autonomy for the sake of curricular coherence. It requires taking action; it may bring long-festering problems to the fore; and it takes time.

It also is quite feasible. Here are some suggestions.

1. It may actually be helpful to be required to respond to mandates from one's professional association, institution, or dean. This, provided that the "push"—as has usually been the case—is not overly prescriptive or cast entirely in the mold of accountability.

2. Put collegiality and collaboration to the service of assessment from the very start. The process of developing a departmental assessment program should model from the beginning the kind of collegial relations toward which one is striving. It may seem obvious that planning requires joint discussion and consensus or strong agreement, short of which obstacles will emerge later if assessment is implemented in a meaningful way. Yet there may be a strong temptation, fostered partly by expediency and the desire to avoid "one more committee," to assign the task to a willing (and probably junior) faculty member or, alternatively, to let faculty's curriculum specializations turn into assessment specializations (i.e., the faculty who teach methods become responsible for assessment in that area). This may produce a well-written report but is not likely to provide a stimulus for meaningful faculty involvement in a "conversation" about student learning.

3. Reaffirm the importance of careful and honest internal evaluation—one of the areas of congruence between academic culture and assessment. Assessment could provide the tools with which to identify and address problems before they become intractable, cause frustration and alienation, and possibly, attract unwanted administrative or bureaucratic attention. Such evaluation should be squarely focused on what students are or are not learning and strategies to effect improvements, not on anyone's "failings." This message is more believable if the important learning goals and assessment procedures are established and agreed upon at the outset without reference to individual instructors—especially if they call for gathering data from individual courses.

4. Minimize the requirements for additional time and effort. Many valuable assessment efforts have made use of secondary analysis of students' course assignments and other "naturalistic" methods. Sampling also has its uses, since it may not be necessary to check on every student's accomplishments, in every area of interest, every year!

5. Link assessment to cognate, ongoing departmental and institutional activities, so as to make it part of the natural cycle of departmental work rather

than an occasional exercise undertaken in connection with periodic reaccreditation. The work of curriculum committees, student advising, and assessment in individual classrooms are good candidates for linkages.[19]

6. Find much needed allies and entry or pressure points by appealing to common values. One of the areas of congruence between academic culture and the new agenda of "assessment as conversation" consists of the values that led faculty into teaching. Some may have forgotten, but at least a nucleus will remember. (It helps, of course, if these values also are affirmed in word and deed by one's institution!)

In calling upon the value of a teaching orientation to promote "assessment as conversation," one must be clear about the fact that "preferences for teaching" may carry different orientations. The task here is to press for a suitable reorientation, while at the same time affirming the common value.

The more traditional teaching orientation, which I have termed "passing on the discipline," emphasizes the professor's knowledge and the student's *opportunity* to learn what the professor has to impart. Good teaching, in this perspective, may mean well-crafted and informed lectures but does not necessarily require equally impressive learning. (Of course, students cannot be absolved from responsibility for their own learning. It is, however, a question of emphasis.) The "learning outcomes orientation" takes its point of departure in a meeting ground between the knowledge and insights of the professor and the students' needs. The professor, therefore, has to assume responsibility not only for "good teaching," as defined traditionally, but also for what the students are actually learning. This reorients the definition of good teaching to include its integral link to learning. In the end, this approach seems to lead naturally to assessment of learning outcomes and the assumption of collective responsibility to ensure that students achieve these outcomes.

7. Finally, there is no magical starting point. Departmental learning goals could provide a logical beginning but so could a review of existing student work, undertaken to gain an empirical sense of students' performance and so begin a discussion of faculty's evaluation and relative satisfaction with such levels of accomplishments. Some departments have been moved to action because they were shown data that demonstrated less than acceptable student performance in fundamentally important aspects of learning. The data were not unexpected; rather, they constituted evidence that could not be refuted or avoided. Others have found an interesting question that could be appropriated by most and thus would provide a starting point for discussion. Ultimately, the point is to begin somewhere. And if what you try does not work, look for another door.

The value of this search, of your work, will be reaffirmed if you bear in mind that the path on which you are engaged can take you to much more important ends than satisfying the National League for Nursing's new accreditation requirements. It leads to the renewed value of one of the most ancient professions—teaching—asserting that a mission to teach is not merely something written on the front page of a college catalogue but is something to be pursued with intensity, dedication, and heartfelt commitment.

NOTES

[1] For a sampling of discussions of the transformation see: on theories of change, Gleick (1987); on organizations, Lincoln (1985); on labor and the international economy, Portes and Walton (1981) and U.S. Department of Labor (1987); on management, Weisbord (1989). With particular reference to higher education, see: on social and cultural diversity, Smith (1989); on the role of higher education in economic development, American Association of State Colleges and Universities (1986); on challenges and new forms of management, Keller (1983).

[2] Real wages peaked in 1973. The median income of individuals declined by 17 percent between 1973 and 1986.

[3] The average annual federal deficit in the 1970s was $33.2 billion. In the 1980s, it was $157.4 billion. During this time, the yearly federal outlay for debt interest doubled, from 10.2 percent to 20.1 percent of all outlays (last figure for 1988). Federal outlays provided 25 percent of state and local budgets in the late 1970s but only 17 percent in 1990. At the same time, new federal mandates required increased state and local spending for social programs (i.e., Medicaid and Medicare especially). The costs of higher education were increasingly borne by students and their families: in 1986, 16.9 percent of college freshmen received Pell Grants, as opposed to 31.5 in 1980; in the same years, the percent of freshmen with GSL loans increased from 20.9 to 25.4.

[4] The assessment movement has made academicians more aware of the importance of stating one's goals in terms of the expected student learning rather than, as was the prevalent practice, in process terms. For instance, "students will be able to apply the major theories of the profession to the practice" (learning outcome goal) rather than "the curriculum provides training in both the theory and the practice of the profession" (process goal). The difference is not merely a semantic one, since the outcome goal involves the responsibility of faculty to help students reach that goal and not just to "exposing" them to relevant knowledge.

[5] At this writing, the future of New Jersey's College Outcomes Evaluation Program is uncertain. The COEP office within the Department of Higher Education has been closed, an action that appears dictated by a combination of the state's fiscal crisis and political considerations.

[6] The decline in the number of 18-year-olds is much more severe in the Northeast and Midwest—ranging from 49 to 30 percent—where 42 percent of all institutions (and 51 percent of private ones) are located (Keller, 1983, p. 12).

[7] The concept of "value added" (later called "talent development") was first put forth by Alexander Astin as a substitute for reputational and resource-based models of institutional excellence (see Astin, 1982).

[8] This is a central point in Rowntree's (1987) book. The author's introduction (p. 1) sets the stage for his approach: "If we wish to discover the truth about an educational system, we must look into its assessment procedures. What student qualities and achievements are actively valued and rewarded by the system? . . . To what extent are the hopes and ideals, aims and objectives professed by the system [actually] . . . striven for?"

[9] Questions about the value of college degrees were prompted mainly by (a) declines in performance on standardized tests: between 1963 and 1979 SAT scores declined by 11 percent in the verbal category and 7 percent in the quantitative. Performance on 11 of the 15 major subject area tests of the Graduate Record Examination also declined between 1964 and 1982. The liberalization of admissions requirements in the 1970s did not explain the decline; and (b) testimony from employers: it was estimated that corporations were spending some $40 billion annually on employee education, much of it in areas considered the responsibility of the educational system.

[10] In 1987, after two years of study, through the College Outcomes Evaluation Program (COEP), the New Jersey Board of Higher Education had mandated outcomes assessment of undergraduate programs in all public colleges and universities. Governor Kean was speaking in the context of resistance to the program from many of the institutions.

[11] As an example of Alverno's use of assessment as learning, students are given the criteria by which they will be assessed and, at each assessment, are asked to apply those criteria to their own performance. Thus self-assessment becomes an integral part of learning.

[12] This work proceeds from the position that, to be most useful, assessment must be close to the everyday work of the faculty. For a description and rationale, see Cross (1988). Cross and Angelo have compiled many procedures—some of them sophisticated and yet quite simple to administer—through which faculty may obtain immediate feedback on student learning in their own classrooms. See Cross and Angelo (1988).

[13] A good, comprehensive overview of the state of assessment, including its purposes, methods, and practices at many institutions is found in Hutchings and Marchese (1990). Other good sources of assessment information are the Assessment Forum of the American Association of Higher Education (Washington, DC) and the Assessment Resource Center at the University of Tennessee at Knoxville.

[14] Portfolios have been "discovered" to be an excellent assessment tool, inasmuch as they provide information on the *growth* of students and can stimulate the conversation about learning. For more information, see Forrest (1990).

[15] For a department to do this, two things are required: (a) a set of common learning goals for the practicum; and (b) departmental discussion, agreement, and, if needed,

training, so that any faculty teaching the practicum will use the same criteria to evaluate students. (This would not prevent faculty from assessing students on their own learning goals in addition to those of the department.) Individual student data, aggregated by goal rather than by student, could then be used to evaluate the curriculum.

[16] My own research with sociology departments lends support to this conclusion, reached by many practitioners. There was an interesting pattern to department chairpersons' answers to the question, "Can assessment help improve how students learn in your department." Answering yes were 21 percent not faced with a mandate; 33 percent planning assessment; 35 percent faced with a mandate; and 46 percent engaged in assessment. The percent replying in the negative was relatively constant (6 to 8 percent in any category); the major shift was from the ranks of the "uncertain" to the ranks of proponents. See Keith & Myers (in press).

[17] These ideas are elaborated further in Keith & Myers (in press).

[18] See, for instance, the theme of the 1987 national conference of the American Association for Higher Education, "Taking Teaching Seriously." Many of the presentations focused on an emerging national agenda for reinserting teaching at the center of academic enterprise. Part of this agenda is a discourse about the "scholarship of teaching."

[19] One connection that should not be made, since it is especially threatening, is that between assessment and the evaluation of faculty for promotion and tenure. The common wisdom is that these two activities should be kept entirely separate.

[20] A list of general reports on secondary and collegiate education up to 1983 is found in the appendix to Integrity in the College Curriculum (AAC, 1985).

REFERENCES

Alverno College (1987). Liberal learning at Alverno. Milwaukee, WI: Alverno College.

American Association of Colleges (1985). Integrity in the college curriculum. Washington, DC: The Author.

American Association of State Colleges and Universities (1986). The higher education-economic development connection: Emerging roles for public colleges and universities in a changing economy. Washington, DC: The Author.

Astin, A. (1982, Spring). Why not try some new ways of measuring quality? Educational Record, 10-15.

Bok, D. (1986). Higher learning. Cambridge: Harvard University.

Boyer, C., & Ewell, P. (n.d.). Glossary of assessment terms. Manuscript distributed at New Jersey Department of Higher Education Assessment Conference.

Clinton, B. (1988). Teaching to rebuild the nation. AAHE Bulletin 40(9), 3-7.

Cross, K. P. (1988). In search of zippers. AAHE BULLETIN, 40(10), 3-7.

Cross, K. P., & Angelo, T. A. (1988). *Classroom assessment techniques: A handbook for faculty*. Ann Arbor, MI: National Center for Research to Improve Postsecondary Teaching and Learning (NCRIPTAL), University of Michigan.

Edgerton, R. (1987). The Spring Hill statement. *AAHE Bulletin, 40*(3), 3–4.

Ewell, P., Finney, J., & Lenth, C. (1990, April). Filling in the mosaic: The Emerging Pattern of State-Based Assessment. *AAHE Bulletin*, 3–5.

Forrest, A. (1990). *Time will tell: Portfolio-assisted assessment of general education*. Washington, DC: Assessment Forum, American Association for Higher Education.

Gleick, J. (1987). *Chaos: making a new science*. New York: Viking.

Groennings, S. (1987). New England in a world economy. *Connection, 1*, 5–10.

Hutchings, P. (1990). Assessment and the way we work. Closing Plenary Address, Fifth AAHE Conference on Assessment (June 30). Washington, DC: The Author.

Hutchings, P., & Marchese, T. (1990, September/October). Watching assessment: Questions, stories, prospects. *Change*, 13–37.

Kean, T. H. (1987). Time to deliver: Before we forget the promises we made. *Change, 19*(5), 10–11.

Keith, N. & Myers, J. (in press). Assessment and undergraduate sociology departments. In S. Sharkey (ed.), *Assessment in sociology*. Washington, DC: American Sociological Association.

Keller, G. (1983). *Academic strategy: The management revolution in higher education*. Baltimore: Johns Hopkins University Press.

Kellogg, J. B. (1988, November). Forces of change. *Phi Delta Kappan*, 199–204.

Lincoln, Y. S. (1985). *Organizational theory and inquiry: The paradigm revolution*. Newbury Park, CA: Sage Publications.

Marchese, T. (1988). Partners in learning: An Interview with Governor Rudy Perpich and Frank Newman. *AAHE Bulletin, 41*(3), 3–6.

Mingle, J. (1989). The political meaning of quality. *AAHE Bulletin, 41*(9), 8–11.

Northeast Missouri State University (1984). *In pursuit of degrees with integrity*. Washington, DC: American Association of State Colleges and Universities.

O'Keefe, M. (1989). Private colleges: Beating the odds. *Change, 21*(2), 11–19.

Portes, A., & Walton, J. (1981). *Labor, class, and the international system*. New York: Academic Press.

Rowntree, D. (1987). *Assessing students: How shall we know them?* New York: Nichols Publishing.

Smith, D. G. (1989). *The challenge of diversity: Involvement or alienation in the academy?* Ashe-Eric Higher Education Report No. 5. Washington, DC: School of Education and Human Development, George Washington University.

U.S. Department of Labor (1987). *Workforce 2000: Work and workers for the 21st century*. Washington, DC: U.S. Department of Labor.

Weisbord, M. (1989). *Productive workplaces: Organizing and managing for dignity, meaning, and community*. San Francisco, CA: Jossey-Bass.

2

Assessing the Goals of Nursing Education: Issues and Approaches to Evaluation Outcomes

Carrie B. Lenburg

Assessment of outcomes has become a central concern in all segments of education and business. Local, national, and international events leave no choice but to deal with generalized incompetence in the work force and the inadequacy of the current educational systems. Before beginning the discussion of technical solutions and the process of outcomes assessment, however we must understand that it is a national, social policy issue and the realization of its purpose requires our collective responsibility in changing conventional perceptions and ways of behaving. A window of opportunity to make a unique contribution to nursing and health care does exist. But to use this opportunity requires that we concern ourselves with something more than individual school, workplace, and personal needs. The National League for Nursing's (NLN) current focus on outcomes assessment is consistent with this broader view in higher education; it is relevant, essential, and, like other major paradigm shifts, requires determination and concerted attention to reach practical fruition.

In this paper, I will provide a comprehensive perspective by reviewing some key points related to the context of the outcome assessment movement, the relationship of concepts and the new criteria for accreditation, some of the concerns and consequences of implementing outcome assessment, and the challenges we face in bringing about essential educational reform based on accountability for competence. I will briefly review various types of evaluation in relation to the new term: *outcome assessment*. Because restrictions of time and space dictate brevity, I invite your thoughtful concentration and commitment to further study.

During the past several years many NLN conferences have focused on the curriculum revolution and the caring curriculum (NLN, 1988, 1989, 1990). The assessment revolution, which some of us started 20 years ago and which is only now being taken seriously, incorporates many of the same components (Lenburg, 1975, 1976, 1979b, 1984, 1990). Both these movements are forcing us to reconsider the fundamental purpose of education and learning, our public accountability, the benefits of collaborative partnerships in the learning process, and the need for authentic relationships in education and practice. These two curriculum trends also contribute to a more holistic movement. We must find ways to integrate them into a comprehensive philosophy and action plan, and focus them to increase competence in learning and practice, in both social and occupational spheres of life, to meet the needs of a society in crisis.

THE CONTEXT

Changes in Society

Comparisons are being made between aspects of U.S. society and those in third world countries. With alarming regularity in daily news broadcasts and other media, the evidence to prove such comparisons is growing. Children grow up experiencing homicides, suicides, substance and person abuse, pregnancy, AIDS, homelessness, poverty, and despair as "normal." Environmental hazards on a local and global scale threaten the world's peoples, including those of us in upper and middle class America, as well as the poor. Lack of health care, inadequate support for education at all levels, escalating school dropout rates, and joblessness characterize large segments of the population and cast ominous shadows on future prospects unless current trends are reversed. As citizens and professionals, nurses can make a difference in this scenario through concerted and collaborative efforts to implement methods that demand competence and encourage caring behaviors in learning and practice.

Economically, the United States is struggling against strong foreign cur-
rents to stay a leader in the global market. With the loss of hundreds of
thousands of jobs more families are added to the poverty statistics and the
cycle of negative conditions just mentioned. Problems associated with the
aging of the population and other demographic changes require a rethinking
of many aspects of health care, learning, work, and leisure. In *Megatrends
2000*, Naisbet and Aburdene (1990) review these and other trends in detail.
Several nurse leaders also have related them to nursing service and education
(Lindeman, 1989; Maraldo, 1990; Moccia, 1989).

These social and economic conditions have a direct influence on nursing
education and nursing service, and we cannot continue to behave as if we are
immune to the need to change. The determination to set reasonable standards
for and to evaluate achievement of outcomes in both education and service is
the beginning point for implementation of reforms essential for survival.

The trend of increasing cultural, racial, and ethnic diversity in the population also bears relevance to the topic of assessment of outcomes. Not only is
such diversity reflected in the student population, but also among coworkers
and recipients of services. It is a three-pronged issue with implications for
curriculum, expected outcomes of learning, and competence in practice. It also
requires an increasing proportion of time and resources for faculty development and curriculum changes.

The insulated and homogeneous culture in which many of us grew up in is
changing rapidly. Many of us from middle America may need to engage in
serious self-reflection about these cultural changes and their consequences
regarding personal myths, biases, and misunderstandings associated with cultural diversity. Only by working collectively and with mutual respect do we
have a better chance of making our multicultural society function harmo-
niously and successfully. As the white majority shrinks in racial terms, more
individuals will become aware that it is not enough to expect that everyone
will acclimate, or be acculturated to, past, stereotypical images of white, middle class, Judeo-Christian America.

As we consider the consequences of these societal changes on education and
health care, and particularly on nursing education, it is easy to understand the
need for essential reforms in instruction and assessment of outcomes for individual students, as well as program and institutional effectiveness. Finding ways
to ensure that students of all types and ages learn required content and are
competent in applying skills related to that content are more critical now than
ever in the history of the profession of nursing. Assessment of effectiveness
begins with identifying desirable goals, ways to get there, and methods to identify when and how we have arrived. This requires a reevaluation of the content,
instructional methods, and competencies considered essential to the profession

both now and in the future. As such, assessment of outcomes at the individual and program levels are both integral to the current reform movement.

If nursing is to be taken seriously as a responsible profession concerned with the public good and capable of participating as a partner in the process of change, its members in the education and service sectors must demonstrate accountability in broad as well as specialized interests. Nurse educators (individually and collectively) will be more effective if they develop a more strategic attitude based on a deeper understanding of significant social and educational changes on a local and national level. It is important, therefore, to comprehend the changes in higher education as part of our context and then to integrate them into nursing education and practice.

Changes in Higher Education: the Assessment of Outcomes Movement

The outcomes assessment movement in higher education is not concerned merely with adding skills tests to the existing academic experience. It is focused on the need for fundamental and far reaching change in all segments and at all levels of education. It is focused on the mission of education to prepare individuals for the work of current and future needs of society, and to ensure competence in the workforce, in the community, and in personal life. It requires a vision for the future, with stated goals, activities to promote achievement of stated goals, and methods to document achievement. Rather than being just another scheme for exerting more policing, requiring more paper work, or exerting more bureaucratic controls for sameness, it is a mechanism to actively shape institutional and program agendas for improving quality of learning. It is concerned with individual course evaluations but only as part of the aggregate abilities of graduates. The assessment movement is directly linked to public accountability, quality of learning in educational institutions, and to demonstrated effectiveness and management of public resources.

Peter Ewell (1990) is a noted authority on outcomes assessment and has written extensively on this subject; the attached bibliography contains a number of publications by him and others, which I urge you to read. Another significant source of information is the annual assessment forum sponsored by the American Association of Higher Education. Proceedings of meetings are available for all five previous conferences.

Basically, legislators, policy-makers, and educators are linking assessment to the "new accountability" and improvements clearly needed in education at all levels. State mandates are being used as incentives for academic institutions to take a long and serious look at the assessment of outcomes as an indicator of quality of education and accountability to the public. Rather than stifling institutional creativity, a competency-based, outcomes-oriented philosophy and approach promote both flexibility and quality.

The U.S. Department of Education and the Council on Postsecondary Accreditation (COPA) also are making changes that require outcomes assessment for accreditation that impact directly on nursing education. COPA is the agency responsible for accrediting NLN and other accrediting bodies, and its mandate was in part responsible for NLN's changes in criteria for accreditation. COPA is exploring two fundamental questions that are particularly relevant for nursing: (1) What is the appropriate relationship of outcomes assessment to accreditation and to institutional and program accountability? (2) What is the accountability of accrediting bodies in the use of outcomes assessment in accreditation? Be on the alert for results from COPA's deliberations.

Changes in accreditation standards are being made to serve the public good through more effective education; the promise of competence is no longer enough. The importance of assessment to accreditation was stated in the Winter 1991 issue of the COPA quarterly newsletter:

> Because accreditation remains the primary and only permanent process within the educational community for assessing and improving educational quality, the accreditation process will directly aid the institutions and programs if it can effectively articulate the role of outcomes assessment in promoting institutional and educational effectiveness.

Changes in Nursing Education

In nursing, trends to require educational effectiveness and public accountability are being stimulated through changes in the criteria for accreditation and the logical extension of these changes into curriculum, expectations for faculty and students, and emphasis on objective evaluation of student outcomes and program effectiveness. Nursing education is subject to the same issues and constraints as all other segments of higher education. How nurses respond to the larger concerns and changes previously mentioned will have very important consequences for our future.

Consider the demographic and cultural changes in the student population in nursing schools and the challenge of teaching for success. The former chairperson of Laguardia Community College's ADN program told me three years ago that students from 28 different countries were enrolled in her program. Golden West College in California has some 1,200 Vietnamese students as well as students from other Asian countries, many of whom are in the nursing program. The barriers for such students are awesome. Many Asian students report that the most important component to being successful in school is the "authentic relationships" they have with caring and helpful instructors.

In addition, the trend of an increasing number of older, experienced working adult learners in nursing education programs has particular relevance to the assessment of outcomes and the consequences of decisions made on the basis of that data. Conventional methods—classroom lectures and other prosaic idioms familiar to most Americans—do not work for persons from nonwestern cultures, especially those whose language, values, and orientations are very different from those of traditional middle-class America. Nor are they effective for working adults whose time is precious and whose primary concerns are often on other issues than repetitive classroom lectures. As we become more sensitive to these significant demographic changes, we also must become more accepting, understanding, and respectful of the talents, background, experiences, perspectives, and insights of these students. By allowing them to become our teachers, we encourage mutual self-esteem and self-efficacy.

What will nursing class profiles look like in five years? in ten years? How will these changes influence education and practice standards, the potential for achieving expected outcomes, and the methods used to evaluate outcomes? The objective assessment of outcomes, for individuals and for programs and services, is needed to spur the implementation of a philosophy of improvement and change in response to the evolving realities of society.

The June 1991 issue of the *American Nurse* reports major efforts by NC-NIP to recruit nursing students from Mexican, Puerto Rican, Dominican, and Cuban American populations. It also reports the growth in numbers of older students entering nursing programs. The Teagle Foundation LPN to BSN project is more than one year old. These are legitimate and worthy efforts to reduce the nursing shortage but with them come new responsibilities. Teachers must discover new ways to promote learning and success among diverse and challenging groups of students, nurses, and clients, especially those considered "high risk" individuals. All of us need to become more sensitive to sharing the responsibility for adaptation and using cultural strengths and diversity to enhance self-esteem and confidence among vulnerable groups. We cannot expect everyone else to accommodate to our status quo. Our beliefs and practices related to evaluation and competence also must take into account the diversity of backgrounds, talents, as well as limitations of students, employees, and clients.

The mandates for outcomes assessment in higher education influence nursing education in several categories. First, the quality of preparation of students entering nursing will affect the success of the faculty and students in meeting their goals. The effectiveness of the outcomes assessment system could make all the difference here. Reforms in instruction and academic support services are designed to improve competence in general education skills for all students, especially for high risk learners (Jones & Watson, 1990). They also are essential to nursing competence. If students entering nursing do not have these skills—reading, thinking, communicating, computing—the nursing faculty will be forced to help such students to learn, or be willing to accept high failure among students who otherwise might have succeeded and contributed to society.

Second, the budgets for nursing programs and the associated human and material resources to accomplish program and the profession objectives are at stake. Nursing education budgets are directly linked to funding of parent institutions; cuts in funding to colleges and universities affect the ability of faculty to provide the kind of educational experiences required to prepare nurses for the sometimes overwhelming, always complex needs of society.

Statewide funding to academic institutions increasingly is being linked with assessment of outcomes as one indicator of accountability. Performance-based funding formulas are being used in several states and assessment is seen more and more as a salient component of the rationale for education budgets. Nurse educators cannot afford to take a passive or reactive attitude toward the funding of their parent institutions; instead, nurse educators must become more actively involved in planning, establishing goals and policies, and in identifying and implementing specific activities directly focused on assessment of outcomes as the mechanism for providing evidence of a willingness to become more responsive to the current and emerging needs of student populations and the society at large.

Third, this is an opportunity for nursing faculty to exert leadership in broader issues related to academic reform, by expediently initiating outcome assessment systems and creating a plan that articulates desired ends and justifies means for achieving them. Information about performance of students, and the program as a whole, should be used proactively. For example, deliberately plan to reveal positive examples and their consequences to policy makers and move them into public awareness. Nurse educators must remember that this faculty reform movement requires conscious involvement from all professionals involved regardless of place on the organizational chart.

Assessment, per se, is not the goal, rather its philosophy and methods force educators to set goals, determine specific plans and activities to accomplish goals, and specify mechanisms for documenting attainment of goals. It is a mechanism to promote broad educational reform and revitalize curriculum. Its specific purposes are: to improve quality of learning and instruction, to increase satisfaction of the learners, and to ensure that graduates are competent to meet the needs of the society in which they will work and live, now and in the twenty-first century. It also is intended to increase accountability among educators and administrators for documenting academic effectiveness and stewardship of public resources.

Determination of quality of education is linked to evidence of satisfactory performance of learners and graduates. This is directly linked to educational content, specific outcome behaviors, and other statements that specifically define competence, consistent with current needs of society and standards of academic and professional agencies and organizations. By focusing on outcomes, the benchmarks of educational effectiveness are less likely to be associated with process-oriented traditions and the quantification of such factors as space, library holdings, class hours, faculty activities (e.g., the number of grants, research projects, and manuscripts produced).

Considered in this context, performance assessment inevitably focuses attention on the learner and activities specifically directed at improving the learner's ability to attain desirable competencies. This means that faculty must specify the skills to be attained, recommend ways for learners to achieve them, and use methods to objectively document competence.

This is not the time to be fearful, uncertain, resistant, or conventional. It is, however, an opportunity to apply the very skills nurse educators require of students and nurses: to be scientifically oriented problem solvers. More precisely, educators need to focus more attention on helping students learn how to learn, to use critical thinking skills based on a broad theoretical base, and to become risk-takers willing to change actions and methods that no longer work both in theory and practice.

The dramatic shifts and trends in society require that we rethink, reconceptualize, and develop a re-vision of the central purpose of nursing education. *Eight-year cycles of repackaging or relabeling the same content, expectations, and traditional methods no longer will suffice.* The focus must expand to incorporate strategies for *learning* as well as teaching and an emphasis on *competence* rather than completion.

THE CONCEPTS AND CRITERIA

Shifting to a new paradigm is confusing until the new concepts, ideas, and methods are related to more familiar doctrine. As we attempt to understand and integrate these new requirements for documenting program effectiveness, think about the following explanation by Marilyn Ferguson in *The Aquarian Conspiracy* (1980):

> *A paradigm shift is a distinctly new way of thinking about old problems. It involves principles that were there all along but unknown to us. It includes the old as a partial truth, one aspect of how things work, while allowing for things to work in other ways as well. By its larger perspective, it transforms traditional knowledge and new observations, reconciling their apparent contradictions. She continues by saying: "we are not so much wrong as partial, as if we had been seeing with a single eye. It is not more knowledge, but a new knowing."*

The shift to a different way of evaluating the quality of educational programs and the merits for accreditation incorporates most of what has been expected all along. The new emphasis, however, provides incentives for educators to return to the true purposes of education (preparation for and competence in work and living) and to a more comprehensive interpretation of achievement (program components and graduate performance). The components fit together very well; they are logically connected and mutually interdependent. One part without the other is inadequate, and until now, the focus and methods of program evaluation have been partial at best. By understanding and integrating the components of the old and new approaches, we can adapt and create a better system of education.

Program Structure, Objectives and Assessment

Figure 2-1 illustrates the broad structural components of a nursing program: administration, faculty, curriculum, and resources. Until 1991, the criteria for approval and accreditation of programs focused on data pertaining to these categories. A school cannot function effectively without them; data related exclusively to them, however, are partial and inadequate. The actual effectiveness of teaching and learning, (i.e., the program) is found in other outcome measures. The program of learning is based on a particular philosophy and statement of overall program objectives that guide the development of courses, classroom, and clinical experiences, and the multiple learning activities that help learners become competent and meet established requirements. These components assume an even greater importance under the new philosophy of outcomes assessment.

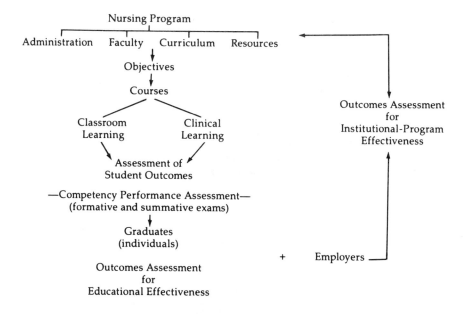

Figure 2-1
Comprehensive Assessment of Outcomes

Educational Effectiveness: Outcomes Assessment

As seen in Figure 2-1, assessment of student outcomes (evaluation) is another major component of the educational program. That it always has been and continues to be important in the learning process and in accreditation criteria merely reinforces its importance. Student outcomes also are directly linked to program and course objectives. In recent years, increasing emphasis has been put on evaluation for a variety of reasons, including the promotion and expansion of both competency based education and adult education movements. Increased precision in developing and using formative evaluation during the learning process and summative examinations to document competence are important faculty activities in improving student learning and preparation for work.

The success of external degree programs based on objective written and performance examinations and procedures also has provided models for the design and use of comprehensive and sophisticated assessment of outcomes for individual learners. These competency based performance assessment methods are crucial in the objective documentation of educational effectiveness at the individual level. In the new outcomes assessment system and under the new criteria for accreditation, instruments designed for specific content and competencies are expected to be used as one kind of measure of quality. When used in combination with external measures they also become significant indicators of the overall program effectiveness (Lenburg, 1984, 1990; Lenburg & Mitchell, 1991; Mitchell, 1987).

Institutional Effectiveness: Outcomes Assessment

Final evaluations of the student's performance at the time of graduation provides the culminating information of internal educational effectiveness, that is, individual student outcomes. These outcome measures, such as comprehensive cognitive and/or performance examinations, also contribute to subsequent assessments for program effectiveness.

The program of learning, the academic support services, faculty efforts, work by the students, and internal means of evaluation are relative. The most significant indicators of success, however, are whether or not the graduate can meet professional expectations. After the student graduates, additional outcome measures are needed to provide salient data on a broader level. Follow-up studies can be designed to determine success on licensure examinations, gaining and maintaining employment, and continued personal and professional development. Surveys and/or interviews of graduates and their immediate supervisors designed to evaluate the effectiveness of the graduate in relation to expectations and the performance of other graduates are potentially the most important measures of program effectiveness.

The new NLN outcome criteria are designed to stimulate the collection of this kind of information with this purpose: to use the data in a deliberate plan to promote improved student learning and competence. The more objective and comprehensive the data, and the more conscientiously they are used, the better the chances are for improving the quality of the program.

Outcomes assessment of program effectiveness, therefore, is determined by a combination of two sets of data: (1) the students' achievement of stated cognitive and performance expectations during and at the conclusion of the program and (2) subsequent outcome indicators such as NCLEX results and performance of graduates after a period of work experience as provided by graduates and supervisors or employers. The major components of the nursing program—the administration, faculty, curriculum, and resources—all influence the achievement of competence of the student and graduate. If graduates do not achieve the objectives, either one or more of these components require revision or the students need more, or a different kind, of assistance.

Analysis of New Outcomes Criteria and BSN Surveys

An analysis of the published outcome criteria for all four councils, summarized in Figure 2-2, indicates similarities and differences in requirements (NLN, 1991). In some categories the interpretation of the criterion is uncertain, pending the development of the suggested or assisting guidelines. The accreditation committees of the councils are meeting and preliminary drafts are expected soon.

As mandated by COPA and the U.S. Department of Education, all four councils include criteria related to graduation rate. The three councils related

Outcomes	BSN	ADN	DI	LPN
General Criteria				
• graduation rate	R	R	R	R
• employment patterns	R	R	R	—
• employer evaluation	O*	O	R	—
• NCLEX results	—	R	R	R
• program satisfaction (graduate satisfaction)	O+	O	R	R
• professional development	O+	O	—	R
ADN and DIPLOMA				
• demographic data	—	O	—	—
• other quantitative data	—	O	R**	—
BSN ONLY				
• critical thinking	R			
• communications	R			
• nursing interventions	R			
• personal development	O+			
• attaining credentials	O+			
• org-work environment	O+			
• scholarship (student/faculty/staff)	O+			
• service (student/faculty/staff)	O+			
• nursing unit defined (unique programs/projects)	O+			

LEGEND

R required	+ use 2 of 8 topics
O optional	* implied
— not cited in material	** standardized tests

Figure 2-2
Comparison of Program Outcomes Assessment Criteria
for Four Education Councils
(Based on preliminary information)

to RN preparation have a specific criterion related to employment rate and patterns; the LPN council does not include it. Only the BSN council does not include a specific criterion related to NCLEX results; however, this may be referenced in forthcoming guidelines. The U.S. Department of Education criteria specifically list inclusion of licensure results where it is applicable. Employer evaluation is optional for BSN and ADN schools and required by the diploma school criteria; it is not mentioned in the LPN criteria. The diploma and the LPN councils specify a criterion for program satisfaction; this is optional for BSN and ADN programs. A criterion on professional development is required by the LPN council, is optional for BSN and ADN programs, and is not mentioned in diploma materials.

The BSN council took a different approach to incorporate outcome criteria by requiring graduation rates and an additional *three student-oriented outcomes*: critical thinking, communication, and therapeutic nursing interventions. They also established a mechanism for flexibility with other criteria, which focus on faculty and staff, the program, and students. Schools are required to select two of eight *optional* areas to use as evidence of program effectiveness. In addition, to the two optional areas already mentioned (program satisfaction and professional development), schools also can select from among the following categories: personal development, attainment of credentials, organization or work environment, scholarship, service, and nursing unit defined.

The Council of Baccalaureate and Higher Degree Programs conducted three surveys of its members related to the specific criteria. In response to the final (March, 1991) survey, approximately 60 percent (376) of BSN programs responded and the overwhelming majority supported the new criteria for accreditation; only three or four respondents were strongly opposed. Under the criterion for program evaluation, ten categories of data for documenting outcomes were specified, as indicated above. Four are required components of evaluation and two others are optional, within a framework of flexibility. Because comparable data were not requested from other councils, comparisons cannot be made.

An analysis of the results provides some insight into the perceived role of nursing programs in relation to graduates and the perceived importance of faculty activities as outcome measures. The rationale for responses was not solicited, but some potential interpretations might suggest topics for further discussion in relation both to criteria for accreditation and methods of outcomes assessment. The magnitude of endorsement may reflect the actual beliefs of faculties and administrators about the purposes of an educational program, priorities among outcomes, and the perceived relative importance of faculty activities and graduate activities as indicators of success.

To present more concise images, the *agree* and *strongly agree* responses are grouped to denote endorsement; all other responses are grouped to denote non-endorsement (including, *neutral, disagree,* and *strongly disagree*). While admitting the dangers of brevity, I suggest that it actually may help us sharpen our focus as we attempt to understand our motivations and beliefs and their relationship to student learning and program outcomes in our own institutions.

As seen in Figure 2-3, five outcome measures are student/graduate focused: graduation rate, professional development, attainment of credentials, employment patterns, and personal development. Two measures, program satisfaction and organization and work environment, are focused on the program. Three additional measures—service, scholarship, and special projects or unit specific activities—are focused primarily on faculty, although graduates also may contribute to the data.

In relation to graduates, only 73 percent of responding schools endorsed completion of the program as a compelling outcome measure of the quality of the program. Approximately two-thirds endorsed professional development, attaining credentials, and employment as essential; they may be saying that these outcomes are generally important, but that the faculty are not accountable. This is very interesting, especially in relation to employment, as the nursing shortage basically ensures a job for any graduate. Although it was not mentioned, passing NCLEX could have been subsumed in this outcome; certification is mentioned. The low endorsement may reflect a collective conviction

OUTCOME MEASURE	NON-ENDORSEMENT	ENDORSEMENT
Graduate		
• GRADUATION	27%	73%
• PROFESSIONAL DEVELOPMENT	32	68
• ATTAINMENT OF CREDENTIALS	35	65
• EMPLOYMENT	36	63
• PERSONAL DEVELOPMENT	58	42
Nursing Program		
• PROGRAM SATISFACTION	16	84
• ORGANIZATION/WORK ENVIRONMENT	36	64
FACULTY		
• SERVICE	14	86
• SCHOLARSHIP	13	83
• SPECIAL PROJECT	19	81

Figure 2-3
**Summary Analysis of BSN Outcome Assessment Measures
(March 1991)**

that attaining credentials is not an important measure for determining the success of the school in preparing graduates for employment and continued education. This is especially puzzling when obtaining licensure is mandatory and certification is either mandatory or strongly recommended for nursing positions. Does this response indicate that faculty think they are not accountable, or that they are fearful of being held accountable for preparing graduates for success?

Another especially sobering and revealing finding is that the majority of respondents did not endorse the outcome of personal development as an essential indicator of the quality of the educational program. At a time of escalating crises in the lives of individuals, families, and communities, this finding seems particularly insensitive to one of the true purposes of education: the preparation of citizens for meaningful and productive lives with a commitment to continued personal and professional development. This outcome measure received the lowest endorsement of the ten listed. On reflection, it seems to reveal an attitude quite contradictory to the recommendations of major higher education commissions as well as the American Association of the Colleges of Nursing (AACN) document, *Essentials of Nursing Education* (1986), a document endorsed by the majority of BSN nurse educators.

The relatively low percentage of respondents who endorsed these outcome measures reflects to some degree the beliefs of faculty and administrators about their roles in preparing graduates for life after college. As faculties begin the process of developing and implementing assessment system, related debates and discussions at the local and national levels will focus and potentially redirect attention on the importance of these outcomes.

In relation to the criterion of program satisfaction, respondents may be indicating that this is important and that they have confidence that graduates will say "good" things about the faculty and the school of nursing; therefore, it is safe to include it. A different perspective is suggested by the response to organization and environment of the school. Only two-thirds endorsed it as a criterion measure of the quality of the program. Could this reflect a lack of understanding of the relationship between these factors and outcomes of learning, of students' success? Or, could it mean that faculty don't want to include it as a requirement because it may reflect poorly in an accreditation report, indicating that the organization and work environment are less than optimum for quality of education? The latter possibility may be influenced by progressive cutbacks in funding with resulting deficiencies in faculty positions, support services, and an environment of frustration with little hope of change in the immediate future. The question, then, is: Does the environment and organization of the school have a significant impact on learning and the competence of graduates to meet expectations of the work world?

All three outcome measures related to faculty received impressive endorsements, quite in contrast to those focused on graduates. Isn't it interesting that faculty activities are valued as more essential outcomes than the graduates' activities? Is this saying that the quality of the nursing program can be determined better by evaluating what the faculty are doing than by evaluating what the graduates are doing? Put another way, the merits and success of the program are validated in *faculty activities more than in graduate accomplishments*. Think about the contrast in regarding physicians here: The competence of a physician is determined by the patient's response to treatment, not the physician's other activities. Shouldn't the competence of the teacher, therefore, be determined by the success of the students and graduates?

THE CONCERNS AND CONSEQUENCES

The Process of Outcomes Assessment

Evaluation always has been difficult. The stakes have just been raised with the advent of the "outcomes assessment movement" in higher education and the changes in NLN accreditation in particular. Changes of this magnitude naturally precipitate some anxiety among educators and administrators. They may even stimulate overt opposition and conflict both within individual programs and at the national level within organizations such as NLN. Current fears, concerns, and conflicts can be overcome by exploring the actual and presumed meanings and consequences of the changes, and by obtaining clarification about the particular points at issue, in addition to actually developing the instruments and processes necessary. In this regard, conferences like this present one and a corresponding series of faculty development workshops are especially useful.

Robert Kirkwood (1981) said: "Assessment has seldom been tried and found difficult; rather it has been found difficult and seldom tried." Circumstances in the society, in education, in health care, in almost every sphere of our living require a revision of the way we conceptualize and activate our beliefs about assessment of the learners' abilities.

Skepticism regarding change is understandable, however, for until recently the gatekeepers and the rules of our professional culture have demanded uniformity and have been resistant to allowing creativity, diversity, flexibility, and even sensitivity to the range of needs of a changing student population. Although such detrimental uniformity and inflexibility seem to be changing, many of us are not quite sure whether or not to really believe this, or what the consequences will be if we do trust in this bold new approach taken, for instance, by "the new NLN."

The surveys on changes in accreditation criteria returned by schools from all councils indicate, at least superficially, that the majority of schools support the changes discussed here generally. Even so, it is probable that most faculties feel concerned about accreditation, how outcome findings will be used, and the consequences of publicly reporting such findings. It also is normal to feel somewhat skeptical about trusting that this new system will be any less frustrating than the previous system. The unspoken fear related to trust is present and needs to be discussed.

Some concerns about outcomes assessment relate to the logistics and purposes of the process. For example:

- Who will do it? Who should be involved in deciding who should be included? Who will develop the instruments? Who will maintain the records, the computer databases? Who will pay for it, especially with increasing budget cuts?
- When and where will it be done?
- How and how often will it be done and through what procedures and with which instruments? To what extent are responses reliable? Can they be trusted in light of their consequences?

Truth and Consequences

Concerns and questions about use of the findings and related consequences are even more troubling. Faculty also may be less likely to discuss these concerns openly. It is essential, therefore, that faculty are targeted for discussion as part of the design of the change process. Some key questions for consideration include:

- What are the consequences of finding out the opinions of graduates and their employers, their degree of satisfaction and recommendations for change? Consider the effects on teachers, administrators, employers, and current and prospective students.
- What are the consequences for relationships among faculty and with students, and between the nursing department and other departments in the institution?

The consequences of reporting the findings to the public and to gatekeeper organizations may be of even more concern.

- How will these revelations affect the school's reputation within the institution and in the community?
- How will the findings influence approval and accreditation by regulatory bodies?
- How will the findings influence potential or actual funding from federal, state, or private sources? Is this another example of governmental intrusion into education, involving more policing and control?
- How will the findings influence marketing strategies, recruitment, and retention of students?
- What influence will the findings have on faculty jobs, salaries, workload, faculty attitudes and behaviors with students, graduates, and peer groups?
- How will the published findings influence the kinds of students admitted into the nursing program in the future?

Other questions are:

- Who is going to interpret the findings and with what perspective or educational philosophy?
- What assurance does a school have that discrimination won't occur against those schools that engage in educational practices different from the norm of the board of review, or site visitors?
- Who will decide the level of acceptability for each outcome criterion?
- What kind of rationale and plan for action will be accepted in relation to the findings of outcomes evaluation?
- How good is good enough to satisfy the board of review?
- What specific measures will emerge as the most desirable for schools to use, even though they are not prescribed in the criteria or guidelines? (What are the unwritten requirements?)
- On what basis should schools trust the site visitors, the board of review members, and the NLN staff any more than in the past?

Trust and Maturity

The leadership and membership of NLN have made some remarkable changes in the evolution of the new criteria and accreditation process. If they are integrated in the spirit as well as the letter of the law, they will ensure more accountability, more effectiveness, and a higher level of trust in the integrity of the system. They are signs of maturity in the profession. The following changes in the accreditation process are examples:

- A restructured decision-making process so that site visitors make initial decision and recommendations to the board of review
- A new kind of orientation for site visitors and board of review members
- Schools recommend faculty for these positions
- At the conclusion of the required orientation for site visitors and board members, both site visitors and board members evaluate each other in a peer review process, against specified criteria. The final and most critical questions are: would you recommend this person? would you want to conduct a program review with this person? and, would you want this person to review your program?
- Moving from very structured criteria that require sameness among schools to a system that deliberately encourages flexibility and adaptations in response to the needs of students being served and the mission of the school.

These changes provide the basis for a new beginning, a new era. Rather than use time and energy focusing on the perceived threats of accreditation, faculties can engage in the more fundamental problems of creating a curriculum that promotes competence among graduates.

On another side of the issue, questions are raised about credibility and standards. For example:

- How can academic and professional standards be maintained with criteria that have no teeth and are so broad and ambiguous as to allow almost any response?
- What can nursing programs use now as a lever with administration to obtain the resources and support for changes needed to improve the program?

·Whenever evaluations are conducted, the potential exists for the results to be used either to benefit or harm the individuals or groups involved, whether students or programs. As part of professional accountability in any change process, we need to anticipate both negative and positive outcomes and to plan in advance the strategies to minimize negative consequences. Our ability to do this successfully will indicate our level of professional maturity.

THE COMMITMENT AND CHALLENGE

The challenge is complex and compelling and can be used to stimulate empowerment for both faculty and students. Some key components are reviewed here as an outline for more detailed subsequent discussions.

44 CARRIE LENBURG

Competence: A Philosophy of Engagement

In its broadest sense, competence is more than a set of behaviors; it is a perspective, a belief system, a philosophy of engagement. It is a way of being, either as teacher or learner. For teachers, it requires modeling the kind of behaviors learners need to learn and acquiring and maintaining competence in clinical practice. It requires keeping informed about changes in the discipline as well as concerns of society at large. It requires having an attitude of engaging in continued learning and setting an example for students and others. It requires a respect for creativity, flexibility, sensitivity, and persistence in helping students to become competent in nursing, particularly if the students are characterized as high risk.

At the core of the assessment movement is the reformation of teaching effectiveness as measured by student learning. Little will be gained from outcomes assessment unless substantive changes are made in the expected roles and the competence of teachers. The attached reference list contains examples from higher education literature that are applicable to nursing. Some are modernized versions of former teaching-learning strategies, such as peer teaching and learning, the use of stories to connect new learning with familiar structures, discussions rather than lectures, exercises to promote critical thinking, and research in the classroom to improve teaching and learning. I recommend that nursing faculty actively engage in learning and applying them in their programs.

Faculty Development: Learning and Change

Like any other major change, administrators, teachers, and others need to implement a plan to promote understanding of outcomes assessment, its consequences, and the reforms needed to promote more effective learning and competence among students and graduates. The change is not fulfilled by conducting follow-up surveys only, but by implementing the philosophy of engagement and the strategies associated with competence of teachers and graduates.

Most faculties will require a period of self-evaluation and planned continuing learning to prepare for these new responsibilities, individually and collectively. A first major hurdle involves overcoming the concerns and resistance to the idea; learning to implement substantive changes in the curriculum that focus on competencies needed in practice and in living is where the actual reform takes place. Program leaders should create a plan and schedule for faculty development, conceived as a long-term period of focused renewal and reorientation of educational mission and philosophy. The plan would help faculty to learn how to implement new teaching-learning strategies and create a system of objective methods to assess competence in essential nursing abilities as well as overall program effectiveness.

Leadership and Involvement

This is a time for assertive and creative leadership and involvement by faculties, administrators, and students. Leaders can help in a number of activities, such as those suggested below.

1. Initiate deliberate occasions for discussions at the local and/or state levels. Assessment methods could be developed collaboratively and shared for cost effectiveness and richness of diversity of thinking. Flexibility, creativity, sensitivity, and persistence are characteristics that describe the process.

2. Avoid the tendency of "regression to the mean" and to the comfort zones where all schools look the same. The same basic principles can be applied differently as needed by the diversity of the student population, the environment, the resources, and the preparation of the faculty.

3. Find ways to avoid the misconception that accreditation and outcomes assessment are police actions and require more paper work. Stimulate the image of reform, for revitalizing the learning process, the creative and empowered capacity of teachers to help learners reach for and achieve their full potential, and for both to become more competent.

4. Deliberately analyze statewide assessment initiatives and apply relevant aspects to your campus and nursing program. Based on this study, implement faculty development activities, initiate plans for the development and implementation of performance assessment systems; reevaluate the meaning and methods of evaluation of students, faculty, and educational support efforts used in your program and institution.

5. Lobby to participate in efforts on your campus or statewide assessment outcomes committees. Demonstrate willingness and readiness to change, to integrate, and even to take leadership in the educational reform movement.

6. Study proceedings from past conferences sponsored by the AAHE, the Assessment Forum, and The Center for Critical Thinking. Read pertinent literature on higher education and non-nursing disciplines

related to assessment and educational reform; attend these forums as part of faculty development strategies.

7. View the new NLN series of videotapes on evaluation as a stimulus for performance assessment component of outcomes assessment.

8. Use expert consultants for specific analysis and adaptations in your school; this is part of long-term faculty and curriculum development strategies.

Dimensions of Evaluating Success

In analyzing the factors that influence individual student success, a constellation of variables emerge as significant. Currently, I am developing a multi-dimensional evaluation framework that includes the following major components:

1. Characteristics of the individual learner
2. Persons who influence success, including those inside and outside the education environment
3. Structures and environment that influence learning, including such factors as the type of curriculum, teaching-learning practices, and policies for individualizing the program of learning
4. Unanticipated life events for student, faculty, and significant others in the learning process.

These factors can be used as components of a program evaluation plan used in conjunction with other outcome measures.

DESIGN AND IMPLEMENTATION OF OUTCOMES ASSESSMENT SYSTEM

During the past few years many schools have implemented some form of assessment of clinical performance. Faculties are learning to apply basic psychometric principles, concepts, and logistics in developing norm-referenced and performance examinations, both for formative and summative evaluation. These forms of assessment are directed to individual learners at various times in the program and are focused on specific competencies and discrete behaviors required for nursing practice. They are essential and integral parts of a comprehensive outcomes assessment plan.

In addition, program evaluation methods must be developed to determine outcomes in the broadest sense. The design and implementation of outcome assessment instruments and analysis of findings require a combination of approaches and considerations used in psychometrics and survey research. Both outcomes assessment of program effectiveness and assessment of individual achievement require clarification of purpose, specificity of questions, objectivity, sampling, consistency, comparability, and established levels of acceptability as essential concepts (Lenburg, 1979a; Lenburg & Mitchell, 1991). Unless individual competencies during the program are achieved it is unlikely that goals for program effectiveness can be met. Thus, the student's achievement of specific competencies and skills is an important component of outcomes assessment. The implementation of the new NLN criteria for accreditation, and those of the regional associations, incorporate both the documentation of success of students/graduates and effectiveness of the program as a whole.

A Proposal: Create An Agenda for Nursing Education Reform

Some major changes recommended at NLN's 1991 convention are included in the document: "Nursing's Agenda for Health Care Reform." At least 42 organizations have endorsed the plan and the profession is about to take some courageous and responsible steps to influence the shaping of health care, not just nursing care. I strongly urge all readers to seriously consider the implications for nursing education, especially our collective responsibility to document that nursing students and practitioners are competent. If the plan is enacted, the need for nursing services will increase and change even further. How should nursing education be modified in anticipation of these changes in service delivery systems, diversity of populations, and settings? What do nurses of the future need to know? How will they be prepared to practice competently, and what systems will be used to hold them accountable?

As an educator reading the document, I substituted the word *learner* in place of the word *consumer*, and the word *education* for *health care systems* and realized that much of what is presented in this document is applicable to the education reform movement. Clearly, the reforms needed in nursing education parallel those outlined in the health care agenda. By paraphrasing some key points, the issues pertaining to nursing education reform are highlighted: We need a restructured education system that enhances learner access to services by delivering educational options in community based settings (making learning experiences more accessible to the working adult learner); one that fosters responsibility for learning and competence among faculty and students; and one that facilitates use of most cost-effective options and settings that differ by population groups and learning objectives.

To help achieve the reforms in nursing education mandated by the outcomes assessment movement, I propose that organized nursing consider developing an *Agenda for Nursing Education Reform*, similar to Nursing's Agenda for Health Care Reforms. To accomplish reforms in health and nursing care, we need nurses who are competent in an array of abilities required for this challenge. As such, we need to undertake a comprehensive reevaluation of nursing education and the changes that need to be implemented to achieve the goals of education for the profession.

The "curriculum revolution" focuses on caring; the "assessment revolution" emphasizes competence; the "agenda for health care reform" emphasizes accountability. The educational reform I propose requires the integration of all three trends into a cohesive and holistic system. This will require vision, leadership, and coordination at the national, state, and local levels. The success of nursing's health care agenda, however, in my opinion, is dependent on fundamental reforms in nursing education already being addressed by competency based performance evaluation and the outcome assessment movement. As the clients of education, students must be given incentives to assume more responsibility for learning and competence. Faculty, functioning as expert consultants, are accountable for helping learners achieve stated objectives. Implementing creative and flexible learning strategies that promote caring and competence and related assessment methods that validate effectiveness in terms of quality outcomes will make substantial contributions to more effective and accountable nursing care delivery as well as better education.

SUMMARY

Oliver Windell Holmes said: "The mind once stretched with a new idea never regains its original dimensions." If we are committed to these new reforms we also are obligated to deliberately learn to change the ways we perceive and implement our roles as educators, researchers, administrators, and clinicians. The client of education (the student), like the client of health care (the patient), must become an active partner and incorporated into the process of change itself. Whether in the service sector or in education, the public is looking for accountability not promises, for competence not just credentials. Those who accept this challenge for change will become revitalized and renewed in purpose, and will be changed, irrevocably.

The essential reforms imbedded in the criteria for evaluation of program effectiveness require that nurse educators successfully undergo a process of reflective, pragmatic, and knowledge-based self-scrutiny designed to reveal deficiencies as well as solutions. Every individual in the profession, at whatever level, has something at stake in this process; working together is one key element to finding solutions. New collaboration and understandings must be reached between those in education and service, between educators and policy makers, between nurse administrators and faculty with counterparts in other disciplines and with institutional administration; and more critically new understandings must be reached in nursing programs of learning: between teachers and administrators, and, at that most fundamental level, between teachers and learners.

We have the knowledge and the vision. As Lucille Joel proudly pointed out in announcing the Health Care Agenda: "Nursing has a new sense of unity of purpose." This plan is not just chipping away at the problem but is taking bold and responsible steps to make the comprehensive changes needed by society. Similarly, the outcome assessment movement in education is another part of taking responsibility for stewardship of public trust and insuring accountability. It is the full implementation of the philosophy of competence, the philosophy of engagement.

Let us stretch our minds to new dimensions and not look back. Let us determine to learn, to change, and not fear what we are capable of learning and doing. It is not an impossible task if we take a long-term view and determine to do it. We will learn to measure the behaviors and outcomes we now find difficult: the affective considerations of caring, critical thinking, moral reasoning, and judgment. We will learn to determine measures of quality of life and patient and student satisfaction. We will learn to integrate competence in high technology with responsive caring about human conditions and health. We will learn to be effective teachers and stewards. The survival of our society, and the life we have known and want for future generations, ultimately, are at stake. Creating and implementing a comprehensive agenda for nursing education reform is a cause worthy of our best and most determined efforts.

SELECTED BIBLIOGRAPHY

American Association of Colleges of Nursing. (1986). *Essentials of College and University Education for Professional Nursing.* Washington, DC: AACN.

American Association for Higher Education. (December, 1990). *AAHE Bulletin* (entire issue: Teaching Learning). Washington, DC: AAHE, 43(4).

American Association for Higher Education. (April, 1990). *AAHE Bulletin* (entire issue: Assessment). Washington, DC: AAHE, *42*(8).

Bevis, E.O. & Watson, J. (1989). *Toward the caring curriculum: A new pedagogy for nursing.* New York: National League for Nursing.

Brookfield, S.D. (1987). *Developing critical thinkers: Challenging adults to explore alternative ways of thinking and acting.* San Francisco: Jossey-Bass.

Claxton, C.S., & Murrell, P.H. (1987). *Learning styles: Implications for improving educational practices.* ASHE-ERIC Higher Education Report No. 4. Washington, DC: American Association of Higher Education.

Conrad, C.F., & Wilson, R.F. (1985). *Academic program review: Institutional approaches, expectations, and controversies.* ASHE-ERIC Higher Education Report No. 5. Washington, DC: Association for the Study of Higher Education.

COPA. (Winter, 1991). *Accreditation: The Quarterly Newsletter of the Council on Postsecondary Accreditation, 16*(1), 1ff.

Cross, K.P., & McCartan, A.M. (1984). *Adult learning: State policies and institutional practices.* ASHE-ERIC Report 1. Washington, DC: American Association of Higher Education.

Ewell, P. (1990). *Assessment and the "new accountability": A challenge for higher education's leadership.* Denver: Education Commission of the States. (Write: Peter T. Ewell, Senior Associate, National Center for Higher Education Management Systems, Education Commission of the States, 707 17th Street, Suite 2700, Denver, Colorado 80202, $5.00)

Ewell, P., Finney, J., & Lenth, C. (April, 1990). Filling in the mosaic: The emerging pattern of state-based assessment. *AAHE Bulletin, 42*(8), 3-5.

Ferguson, M. (1980). *The Aquarian conspiracy: Personal and social transformation in the 1980s.* Los Angeles: J.P. Tarcher, Inc.

Gamache, R.D., & Kuhn, R.L. (1989). *The creativity infusion: How managers can start and sustain creativity and innovation.* New York: Harper and Row.

Grant, G. & Associates. (1979). *On competence.* San Francisco: Jossey-Bass. (Especially: Grant, G., & Kohli, W. Contributing to learning by assessing student performance (138-159); Elbow, P. Trying to teach while thinking about the end, (95-137).

Haddon, R.M. (January, 1990). An economic agenda for health care, *Nursing & Health Care, 11*(1), 21-26.

Hutchings, P. (April, 1990). Learning over time: Portfolio assessment. *AAHE Bulletin, 42*(8), 6-8.

Hutchings, P., & Marchese, T. (1990). Watching assessment: Questions, stories, prospects. *Change, 22*(5), 12-38.

Jones, D.J., & Watson, B.C. (1990). *"High risk" students in higher education: Future trends.* ASHE-ERIC Higher Education Report No. 3. Washington, DC: The George Washington University School of Education and Human Development.

Kirkwood, R. (1981). Process or outcome: A false dichotomy. In *Quality: Higher education's principal challenge,* (T.M. Stauffer, Ed). Washington, DC: American Council on Education.

Kurfiss, J.G. (1988). *Critical thinking: Theory, research and possibilities.* ASHE-ERIC Higher Education Report No. 2. Washington, DC: American Association of Higher Education.

Lenburg, C.B. (1979a). *The clinical performance examination: Development and implementation.* New York: Appleton-Century Crofts.

Lenburg, C.B. (1990). Do external degree programs really work? *Nursing Outlook, 38*(5), 234-238.

Lenburg, C.B. (1979b). Emphasis on evaluating outcomes: The New York regents external degree program, *Peabody Journal of Education, 56*(3), 212-221.

Lenburg, C.B. (1975). *Open Learning and career mobility in nursing.* St. Louis: C.V. Mosby.

Lenburg, C.B. (1984). Preparation for professionalism through regents external degrees, *Nursing & Health Care, 5*(6), 318-325.

Lenburg, C.B. (1976). The promise fulfilled: The New York regents external degree program in nursing. *Nursing Outlook, 24*(7), 422-429.

Lenburg, C.B., & Mitchell, C.A. (1991). Assessment of outcomes: The design and use of real and simulation nursing performance examinations. *Nursing & Health Care, 12*(2), 68-74.

Lindeman, C.A. (January, 1989). Curriculum revolution: Reconceptualizing clinical nursing education. *Nursing & Health Care, 10*(1), 23-28.

Maraldo, P.J. (January, 1990). The nineties: A decade in search of meaning. *Nursing & Health Care, 11*(1), 11-14.

Meyers, C. (1986). *Teaching students to think critically: A guide for faculty in all disciplines.* San Francisco: Jossey-Bass.

Mezirow & Associates. (1990). *Fostering critical reflection in adulthood: A guide to transformative and emancipatory learning.* San Francisco: Jossey-Bass.

Mitchell, C.A. (1987). Future view: Nontraditional education as the norm. In *Patterns in nursing: Strategic planning for nursing education,* New York: National League for Nursing, 71-89.

Moccia, P. (January, 1989). 1989: Shaping a human agenda for the nineties: Trends that demand our attention as managed care prevails. *Nursing & Health Care, 10*(1), 15-17.

Naisbitt, J., & Aburdene, P. (1990). *Megatrends 2000: Ten new directions for the 1990's.* New York: William Marrow and Co.

National League for Nursing. (1990). *The curriculum revolution* (video tape). New York: National League for Nursing.

National League for Nursing. (1988). *The curriculum revolution: Mandate for change.* New York: National League for Nursing.

National League for Nursing. (1989). *The curriculum revolution: Reconceptualizing nursing education.* New York: National League for Nursing.

National League for Nursing. (1990). *The curriculum revolution: Redefining the student teacher relationship.* New York: National League for Nursing.

National League for Nursing. (1987). *Educational outcomes: Assessment of quality—An annotated bibliography.* New York: National League for Nursing.

National League for Nursing. (1987). *Educational outcomes: assessment of quality — A directory of student outcome measurements utilized by nursing programs in the United States.* New York: National League for Nursing.

National League for Nursing. (1990–1991). *Evaluation* (a three part videotape series). New York: National League for Nursing.

National League for Nursing. (1991). *Proposed accreditation criteria changes* (materials from the councils for Associate Degree Programs, Baccalaureate and Higher Degree Programs, Diploma Programs, and Practical Nurse Programs). New York: National League for Nursing.

Paul, R. (1990). *Critical thinking: What every person needs to survive in a rapidly changing world.* Rohnert Park, CA: Sonoma State University, Center for Critical Thinking and Moral Critique.

Schon, D.A. (1983). *The reflective practitioner: How professionals think in action.* New York: Basic Books.

Seymour, D.T. (1988). *Developing academic programs: The climate for innovation.* ASHE-ERIC Higher Education Report No. 3. Washington, DC: Association for the Study of Higher Education.

Smith, D.G. (1989). *The challenge of diversity: Involvement or alienation in the academy?* Report No. 5. Washington, DC: The George Washington University, School of Education and Human Development.

Waters, V. (1989). Transforming barriers in nursing education. In *The curriculum revolution: Reconceptualizing nursing education.* New York: National League for Nursing, 91–99.

Whitaker, U. (1989). *Assessing learning: Standards, principles, and procedures.* Philadelphia: Council for Adult and Experiential Learning.

Whitman, N.A. (1988). *Peer teaching: To teach is to learn twice.* ASHE-ERIC Higher Education Report No. 4. Washington, DC: Association for the Study of Higher Education.

Wright, B.D. (1990). But do we know it'll work? *AAHE Bulletin, 42*(8), 14–17.

3

Program Evaluation in Nursing Education: Creating a Meaningful Plan

Catherine A. Bevil

Systematic program evaluation is an integral component of contemporary educational systems. It is not only expected but demanded by a variety of individuals and groups who have a stake in the educational process, including consumers and other beneficiaries of educational programs as well as those who develop, implement, manage, fund, and accredit programs.

Commitment to systematic program evaluation began shortly before World War I and was directed at programs in education and public health. In the 1930s and 1940s, program evaluation efforts accelerated when social scientists advocated the application of social research methods to the assessment and evaluation of community based programs. The federal government provided an important impetus for expansion of program evaluation projects in the 1950s and 1960s when it committed significant funds to the support of large scale education and community efforts that included an evaluation component (Guba & Lincoln, 1989). The early knowledge base of evaluation, which

The author thanks Charles A. Maher, PhD, Professor and Chair, Graduate School of Applied and Professional Psychology, Rutgers, The State University of New Jersey, Piscataway, New Jersey, and the Program Evaluation Task Force for their assistance on this project.

borrowed heavily from existing methods and theories, has matured and diversified in response to experience doing evaluation (Shadish, Cook, & Levitow, 1991) and affords those involved in evaluation of nursing education programs a rich array of resources on which to draw.

Program evaluation has been an essential part of nursing education for decades. In recent years, however, we have been challenged to expand the scope of our program evaluation activities and enhance the sophistication of our evaluation designs to assure that program evaluation information is comprehensive, meaningful, and useful. The National League for Nursing (NLN), through its accreditation activities, has been an important force in challenging us to enhance program evaluation efforts. A review of the past several editions of the criteria for the evaluation of nursing programs indicates an expansion in focus from evaluation of curriculum plans and processes to evaluation that incorporates all essential program elements and includes outcome evaluation with process evaluation.

Although program evaluation activities have become routine in nursing programs, faculty continue to have questions about how best to plan and implement program evaluation. In addition, many faculties are currently taking another look at their program evaluation plans and making modifications to assure that they incorporate the new emphasis on program outcomes advocated by the National League for Nursing.

PURPOSE

In this paper, I will describe a project to develop and implement a comprehensive program evaluation plan within a department of nursing in a university health sciences center. I will describe the phases of the program evaluation planning process being used and I will discuss strategies found helpful during the planning process. These strategies allow the program evaluation process to be tailored to fit the unique characteristics, strengths, and values of the nursing program, thereby promoting success of program evaluation activities. It is hoped that this paper will stimulate thinking about effective ways to structure the process of creating a meaningful program evaluation plan.

BACKGROUND

This project began at Thomas Jefferson University in early 1989 when Dr. Pamela G. Watson, chairman of the department of nursing, and the faculty recognized that the existing program evaluation plan no longer met the needs of the department which had undergone rapid expansion. Within a few years, additions had been made to the initial generic baccalaureate program including a baccalaureate completion program for RN students, a master's degree program, and a part-time evening curricular option within the full-time generic baccalaureate program. The chairman's goal was creation of a comprehension evaluation plan that fully encompassed the department's expanded purposes and activities and would serve the department in decision making, planning, and development now and in the future. Achieving this goal would require that all faculty in the department understand the purposes program evaluation could serve and be committed to making program evaluation a part of department routine. Early on, it was recognized that the project would be a major undertaking that would require careful planning and a special investment of time and departmental resources.

CHARACTERISTICS OF AN EFFECTIVE PROGRAM EVALUATION PLAN

If a program evaluation plan is to serve decision making, development, and planning, it must possess several characteristics, including practicality, utility, propriety, and technical adequacy. Practicality means that a program evaluation plan is both feasible and usable. An evaluation plan must be implemented as a routine programmatic activity throughout the academic year. From a pragmatic standpoint, however, implementation should not disrupt other important nursing program activities. Furthermore, the cost of implementing program evaluation on an ongoing basis in terms of time and financial and human resources should be within the budgetary guidelines of the nursing program. Second, a program evaluation plan should be useful. An evaluation plan should be able to provide evaluation information that clearly documents the effectiveness of the nursing program and is helpful to faculty in developing and improving the program. Propriety, the third characteristic, refers to the need for methods, instruments, and procedures included in the evaluation plan to adhere to all legal and ethical standards. The final characteristic is technical adequacy. Instruments and procedures used to collect and analyze evaluation data need to possess levels of validity and reliability that are acceptable to all those involved in the evaluation process, particularly those who will be using the evaluation results. Development of a program evaluation plan that possessed these four characteristics was our goal throughout the planning process.

ASSURING SUCCESSFUL PROGRAM EVALUATION

As the planning process continued we identified several broad strategies that have helped to assure a successful outcome: (1) identifying and using a theoretical or conceptual base to guide the evaluation process; (2) tailoring program evaluation activities to fit the program's existing organizational structure, governance, and routine practices; and (3) capitalizing on the program's existing human and material resources.

Using a Theoretical Base

Using a theoretical or conceptual approach to guide the evaluation process helps assure that the plan that is developed is both comprehensive and coherent. The field of program evaluation, including its definitions, purposes, methodologies, theories, and models, has undergone refinement and expansion, especially in the past three decades. Many program evaluation models are available to use in their entirety or in modified form when developing a program evaluation plan.

After reviewing the literature, our faculty concluded that no one contemporary evaluation model incorporated all the concepts they wished to use. As a result, we adopted an eclectic model that includes concepts from classic evaluation models (Popham, 1974; Provus, 1971; Roth, 1978; Stake, 1967; Stufflebeam, et. al., 1967; Tuckman, 1967; Worthen & Sanders, 1973) as well as newer concepts of evaluation, particularly those of the responsive constructivist model developed by Guba and Lincoln (1989). Our model includes a definition of program evaluation that specifies its purposes and processes and includes a framework for describing and analyzing an educational program. Using this framework assured that the scope of our evaluation was comprehensive. Our model also incorporates mechanisms for generating meaningful evaluation questions and for making evaluation decisions. Selected elements of our evaluation model are outlined in Table 3-1.

Our evaluation model has been helpful in directing the phases of the evaluation planning process (see Table 3-2). The phases of the planning process, as we have experienced them, include: (1) analyzing the program to place it into an "evaluable" program form; (2) identifying meaningful evaluation questions; (3) constructing program evaluation protocols to answer each evaluation question; (4) field testing and revising evaluation methods, instruments, and procedures; and (5) finalizing the evaluation plan. In a later section of this paper, I will describe each of these phases in more detail and in relation to our evaluation model.

Table 3-1
Selected Elements
of an Evaluation Model

Defining Program Evaluation:
  –Scope
  –Purposes
  –Process
  (Stufflebeam et al., 1971)

Analyzing the Nursing Education Progam: The CIPP Model
  –Context
  –Input
  –Process
  –Product
  (Stufflebeam et al., 1971)

Generating Meaningful Evaluation Questions:
  –Surveying Stakeholders
  (Guba & Lincoln, 1989)

Making Evaluation Decisions:
  –Using Standards
  (Provus, 1971; Stake, 1967)

Table 3-2
Phases of the Program Evaluation Planning Process

1. Conduct an analysis of the program to place it in an "evaluable form"
2. Generate meaningful evaluation questions
3. Construct evaluation protocols to answer each question
4. Develop, field test and revise evaluation instruments, methods and procedures
5. Finalize the program evaluation plan

Tailoring Activities to Existing
Structure and Governance

We believed that success in making the significant changes required by a new evaluation plan would be more likely if both the planning process and the final evaluation plan were consistent with other already accepted and successful mechanisms for conducting business within the department. Therefore, we tailored our planning activities as well as the methods and procedures prescribed in our evaluation plan to the department's existing structure and governance. These had undergone recent revisions designed to facilitate the work of the department.

Our bylaws do not include a standing committee charged with evaluation activities and the faculty did not view the establishment of one as necessary. However, since the bylaws provide for the formation of task forces to accomplish discrete, short-term projects, the Program Evaluation Task Force was established to develop the evaluation plan. Although task force membership was voluntary and open to all individuals who held faculty rank, efforts were made to assure that its membership included faculty representation from the several diverse educational programs and constituencies within the department.

As the program evaluation plan was developed, processes of data analysis, data interpretation, and decision making that were delineated have been designed to capitalize on the existing standing committee structure identified in our bylaws. Each standing committee will assume responsibility for interpreting data, making decisions, and taking action in those areas that pertain to its existing charge. For example, our Student Affairs Committee will oversee evaluation activities relevant to student policies and procedures and our Curriculum Affairs Committee will assume responsibility for evaluating student learning outcomes. We will need to make only minor revisions in our bylaws to assure that relevant program evaluation activities are incorporated in the charge for each of our standing committees.

Long-term success of program evaluation requires the commitment and involvement of those individuals who hold administrative responsibilities in the organizational structure. In our case, the department chairman was already familiar with program evaluation and valued it. She assured that accountability for program evaluation was built into the formal role responsibilities of the department's program directors and then took steps to recruit individuals to these positions who also understood and valued program evaluation.

Success not only requires the support of individuals with administrative responsibilities within the organizational structure, but demands involvement of all other faculty. Because the specific needs, concerns, and values of each faculty group are different, strategies appropriate for obtaining faculty support will vary accordingly. Assessing the faculty's knowledge of and attitudes toward program evaluation and their previous experience with it provides useful background information when identifying strategies to garner faculty support and involvement. The faculty may need basic information about the program evaluation process and reassurance to dispel anxieties that program evaluation means "personnel evaluation." To introduce faculty to the program evaluation process we tapped the department's existing communication channels, which included planned presentations held in conjunction with monthly faculty meetings, all-day workshops, and dissemination of written materials using existing mechanisms.

Capitalizing on Existing Human and
Material Resources

If a program evaluation plan is to succeed as a part of the daily routine, it needs to capitalize on the human and material resources already available. If budget allows, special expenditures during the planning process to supplement existing resources in areas of weakness can be helpful. The long-term goal is development of a plan that, when implemented over time, will not drain the resources of the nursing program.

For example, we hoped to capitalize on our strength in computer resources by devising a plan that would involve data tabulation and analysis by computer. Most of our faculty possess computer competencies, and the department employs staff specifically designated to facilitate computer utilization. All faculty and staff in our department have office computers. Software available to use includes Lotus, SPSS, and SAS. When selecting computer software for use in our program evaluation activities, we applied the principle of pragmatism and chose the software that was most widely available and accepted within our university. Lotus will be used to visualize statistics in table form and SAS will be used to analyze data from our evaluation questions. SAS will allow analysis of both numeric and alphanumeric data. Sophisticated computer resources, however, are not a prerequisite for a high quality, useful program evaluation plan. Excellent program evaluation plans that yield valid and reliable information can be developed to fit whatever resources a program possesses for tabulation and analysis of evaluation data.

Because few faculty in the department had participated in program evaluation or viewed themselves as comfortable with it when this project was initiated, the department chairman made the decision to supplement faculty expertise in this area and hire an outside consultant to guide the planning process. We have used a consultant in program evaluation through all phases of planning. The author, the first consultant who was selected, is a nurse educator who was familiar with the literature on program evaluation and possessed experience in developing program evaluation plans in other nursing education programs. After this individual was employed as a full-time faculty member in the department, a second consultant was hired who is not a nurse, but who possesses complementary skills including a wealth of technical expertise in all phases of the program evaluation process and competence in computerizing program evaluation plans.

Utilization of an expert consultant in program evaluation should be given serious consideration if a nursing education unit has financial resources that can be committed to one. Depending on the program's budget, the role of the consultant can expand or contract. As an expert in the field, the consultant can be used to increase faculty knowledge about program evaluation and promote positive attitudes about it. Second, a consultant can supply objectivity about the program and its evaluation that faculty do not have. Additionally, the consultant can serve as a guide from the beginning to the end of the project, keeping activities focused and assuring that the planning group adheres to its timetable. If carefully chosen, a consultant can provide expertise in areas the faculty do not possess, assuring that all necessary skills are available for successful completion of the plan.

THE EVALUATION PLANNING PROCESS

We defined program evaluation as "the systematic, cyclical and continuous process of delineating, gathering, and analyzing data about all program elements and using the information for the purposes of decision making about the worth of the program and enhancing program quality and effectiveness." Our definition includes both formative and summative evaluation activities. It also prescribes a comprehensive evaluation, that is, one that incorporates all program elements.

Analyzing The Program

The first step in our planning process was to conduct a comprehensive analysis of the program to place it in an "evaluable" form that would assure inclusion of all program elements. To assist in a systematic and complete program analysis, we selected Stufflebeam's Model (Stufflebeam et al., 1971), which proposes four types of evaluation: context, input, process, and product.

Context evaluation examines the program's mission, purposes, and objectives and determines whether the environment of the program supports the program's purposes and objectives and is conducive to its success. The context (environment) of a program is examined for unmet needs and problems as well as untapped opportunities. For an established program, context evaluation is used to decide whether the initial program planning decisions are still relevant or whether they should be changed to meet changing conditions. The focus of context evaluation is on the program's intended outcomes.

Input evaluation, which focuses on the intended means of the program, also delineates resources available to the program and assesses policies, procedures, strategies, and plans for resource utilization to reach intended goals and objectives. Resources or capabilities to be considered might include students, faculty, curriculum plans, organizational structure and governance plans, policies and procedures, physical resources, facilities and services, and financial resources. Input evaluation deals with the feasibility of achieving goals and objectives given available resources, examines alternative strategies for reaching objectives, and assesses costs and benefits of planned strategies.

Process evaluation focuses on the actual means or procedures in place. Once program objectives and a plan to reach those objectives are developed, process evaluation aims to monitor the implementation of the planned program. It serves implementation functions in controlling the actual operations of the program, determining if the program is being implemented as planned, identifying barriers in implementing the program as planned, pinpointing flaws or deficits in the planned program and providing a record of actual events.

Product evaluation is concerned with the actual outcomes of the program. Product evaluation involves measuring the extent to which program purposes and objectives have been met on a regular basis during and at the end of the program. Product evaluation often involves operationally defining objectives, measuring the attainment of objectives, and comparing the attainment against selected criteria. Product evaluation should focus on both immediate program objectives and long-term program impact. It should encompass both intentional outcomes and side effects. Findings of product evaluation lead to decisions to maintain or modify other relevant areas of the program including its objectives, design, or implementation.

Generating Evaluation Questions

A thorough program analysis serves as the basis for moving to the second phase of the evaluation process, the identification of meaningful evaluation questions. We defined a meaningful evaluation question as one that, when answered accurately, possessed four characteristics: (1) it reflects the claims, concerns, or issues of one or more program stakeholders; (2) it provides information that can be useful to stakeholders; (3) it allows judgments to be made about the worth of one or more program elements; and (4) it provides data that guide and direct faculty in developing and improving the quality of the program.

Because we hoped to develop an evaluation plan that would be relevant to those who had an interest in the program, we incorporated the concept of "stakeholder" into our evaluation model for use at this phase. According to Guba and Lincoln (1989), a stakeholder is any person or group who uses program evaluation data and who, therefore, might be put at some risk by program evaluation. If program evaluation is to be relevant to stakeholders, then their claims, concerns, and issues need to be identified and incorporated into evaluation questions. A claim is an assertion that is favorable to the educational program; a concern is an assertion that is unfavorable to the program; an issue is any state of affairs about which reasonable people might disagree. Different stakeholders have different claims, concerns, and issues. Guba and Lincoln have identified three groups of stakeholders: (1) agents, a broad group including persons involved in sponsoring, producing, or implementing the program (such as faculty, funding agencies, accreditors, and staff); (2) beneficiaries, or individuals who are direct or indirect targets or markets for the program (such as students, parents, and patients); and (3) victims, individuals who are affected negatively because of the educational program but who may not know they are victims. Using this description of stakeholder, we identified the following stakeholders as being especially important: faculty, students, administrators, alumni, employers, clients, funding agencies, and accreditors and other reviewers.

Although it may be beyond a program's available resources to incorporate the claims, concerns, and issues of all stakeholders into an evaluation plan, the views of major stakeholders can be identified and considered. Assuring that claims, concerns, and issues of stakeholders are incorporated in evaluation questions can be accomplished in many ways. These include reviews of literature and other relevant documents, interviews, mail questionnaires, and inclusion of representatives of stakeholder groups in the evaluation planning process. For example, published guidelines are available that provide useful information about the claims, concerns, and issues of funding agencies, accreditors, and other outside reviewers. It was especially important to our faculty that evaluation questions fully incorporate the National League for Nursing Accreditation Criteria.

Stakeholder groups, or relevant samples of them, can be surveyed using an open-ended questionnaire format to identify topics or issues they believe to be important to include in evaluation questions. We believed it was important to survey all our full- and part-time faculty. Interestingly, the evaluation concerns of our faculty primarily reflected the program elements of process and product. Over 60 percent of the faculty's evaluation concerns were categorized as process and less than 30 percent as product. We also surveyed a sample of our student body, who include over 300 individuals. Students were contacted during a course on professional issues to assure that they had sufficient information about the program evaluation process to participate knowledgeably in this activity.

Surveying students as a part of a required class activity also assured that we received a very high response rate from our students.

A mail questionnaire to a representative sample of alumni is another useful mechanism for obtaining information about alumni evaluation concerns. Employers of the program's graduates might best be queried by a telephone survey. This can minimize the amount of time that these individuals need to spend on this activity while assuring a reasonable response rate. All evaluation concerns that are generated by stakeholders can be examined and then transformed, whenever appropriate, into evaluation questions that are clearly and concisely stated.

In addition to developing evaluation questions that were relevant, we wanted to assure that the questions were comprehensive; that is, that they reflected all elements of the program. As questions were generated, each was categorized according to the program element or evaluation type (context, input, process, or product) it most closely reflected. Questions were then reviewed to assure that all program elements were sufficiently represented. The evaluation questions that we developed reflect Stufflebeam's four types of evaluation and address all but a few program elements. For example, our evaluation questions do not address the topic of individual or personnel performance because the focus of program evaluation is on the aggregate rather than the performance of any one individual. In addition, our evaluation plan does not address areas of the program for which authority to make changes lies outside the faculty group conducting the evaluation. These areas include compensation and benefits and professional association and union business.

During this phase of the program evaluation planning process, more than 60 evaluation questions were proposed. Some examples of evaluation questions that were generated are:

To what extent do RN-BSN graduates exhibit professional behaviors different from entry behaviors?

What has been the attrition rate for students? How does attrition relate to admissions characteristics?

To what extent are graduates prepared to meet contemporary demands of nursing practice?

Constructing Evaluation Protocols

The next phase involved the painstaking task of constructing an evaluation protocol to answer each evaluation question. Table 3-3 identifies the six components of our evaluation protocols. Protocols were developed by the

Table 3-3
Elements of an Evaluation Protocol

1. Clear, concisely stated question
2. Variables on which data are collected to answer the question
3. Methods, instruments, and procedures for data collection on all variables
4. Methods and procedures for data analysis and interpretation
5. Personnel, responsibilities, and timelines
6. Guidelines for communication and use of evaluation information

department's evaluation consultant and then critiqued by Program Evaluation Task Force members. This feedback has been essential in revising the protocols to assure they are complete, accurate, and relevant. Refer to Table 3-4 for an abbreviated form of one of our evaluation protocols.

Each evaluation question was analyzed to identify all variables on which data needed to be collected to answer the question completely. Variables were studied to determine the most appropriate method of data collection and the stakeholder groups from whom data should be collected. The protocols prescribe several different methods to collect data about variables, however, the survey instrument is the most common. In most cases, our data collection instruments include a five-point scale and space for open-ended comments after every item. The respondent is usually required to provide a comment in the form of a rationale or example after each item, thus providing meaningful information for use during the interpretation phase of the evaluation process. Sampling is used to collect data from most constituencies, including faculty and students. Sampling will limit the amount of time any one individual must spend on evaluation activities and will help to keep the volume of data collected to a manageable level.

Many protocols specify the use of descriptive statistics to analyze data. Our evaluation plan indicates that student data will be analyzed separately for each of our four student populations because we expect there may be important differences among these groups. Because we have a new evening generic program, we are especially concerned about examining the data that are generated by our evening students. This has been accomplished in two ways. First, their responses on all items will be analyzed separately from the responses of day generic students. In addition, our program evaluation plan includes a significant number of questions that specifically address evaluation of our evening nursing program.

Whenever appropriate, our existing standing committees will be involved in interpretation of evaluation data thereby assuring faculty involvement

Table 3–4
Evaluation Protocol

To What Extent Are the Physical Facilities Adequate for The Nursing Unit to Accomplish Its Goals?

Data Collection Variables

* Adequacy of the physical facilities for academic instruction, college laboratory, and clinical experiences of nursing students at baccalaureate and master's levels, based on judgments of nursing faculty and students.
* Adequacy of physical facilities to support research, scholarship, professional and community service.

Data Collection Methods, Procedures, Instruments

1. Representative samples of nursing faculty at both the baccalaureate and master's levels (n = 10) and representative samples of students (n = 10), in each of four categories (day generic, evening generic, RN-BSN, and Masters) are provided a copy of Instrument 6, NURSING DEPARTMENT PHYSICAL FACILITIES ADEQUACY OPINION SURVEY.
2. Each respondent is asked to use his/her personal experiences in classroom, college laboratory and clinical work in completion of Instrument 6.
3. Each respondent can be given a copy of Instrument 6 in his/her Departmental mail box, with a specific date for return of the completed instrument to the respective Program Director.

Methods and Procedures for Data Analysis and Interpretation

1. Similarities and differences in responses between faculty and students in each of four categories are compared for each item of Instrument 6, using means and other appropriate descriptive statistics.
2. The Department's physical resources can be considered as being adequate overall, if 75% or more of the mean responses per item indicate adequacy or greater than adequacy.

Personnel, Timelines, Responsibilities

1. Instrument 6 is distributed during the spring semester of every other academic year by both Program Directors.
2. Results of survey are disseminated to Faculty Affairs Committee for final decisions on adequacy/inadequacy.

Communications and Use of Evaluation Information

1. Recommendations for change are forwarded to the Chair. Report of action taken to be generated within three months to committee.

through all phases of the evaluation process. Each protocol identifies the committee, group, or individual responsible for interpreting data. Groups will convene with relevant data, dialogue about the meaning and implications for the program, and make recommendations to the administrator or other individual or group identified in the protocol as responsible for decision making in the area being evaluated.

Using standards for data interpretation is an important component of each evaluation protocol. Our definition of standards reflects the work of Provus (1971) and Stake (1967). Standards are the alternatives against which evaluation data are compared. They are defined as "what should be." Standards are based on knowledge, experience and values and are determined by program faculty, administrators, staff, and others who possess the professional expertise to determine appropriate ones. Standards will provide a reference point against which our findings can be compared when making decisions about the quality of a particular program element. As our data pool grows and we learn more about the phenomena we are studying, we expect our standards to undergo revision.

Each protocol also identifies the individual with overall accountability for implementing it. In most cases, this responsibility rests with an individual, such as a program director, with administrative responsibilities in the department. The task of initiating protocols and compiling data will be assigned to a secretary in the department and comprise one component of the secretary's job responsibilities.

Care was used in determining the timetable for evaluation, again to assure that evaluation activities did not become overwhelming. Data collection for the many protocols is staggered throughout the academic year. Although some protocols prescribe data collection annually, others require data collection once every three or four years. When making decisions about the timeline, factors that were considered included the frequency that an area was expected to change and the overall importance of the area within the total program.

Developing Instruments, Methods and Procedures

Once all program evaluation protocols have been developed, data collection instruments can be finalized. It is possible to incorporate two or more protocols into one instrument thereby streamlining the data collection process. Although we have over 60 evaluation questions, each with its own protocol, the number of evaluation instruments is fewer. Each item on every data collection instrument is coded numerically so that it can be traced back to the appropriate protocol and evaluation question. As instruments are developed, they are distributed to a small number of selected respondents, such as faculty and students, for field testing. Based on feedback received, instruments and procedures are revised.

Finalizing the Plan

We expect to complete the planning process and have all instruments in final form by mid-autumn 1991. As a final step, the program evaluation plan will be placed in book form and on computer diskette and available to all those who have a role in the evaluation process.

We have discovered that the program evaluation process does not consist of tidy steps but is a fluid process that involves moving back and forth between phases as the situation requires. Even now we are continuing to add new evaluation questions as phases of the project near completion in other areas. We believe that the investment we have made in planning for evaluation will serve us well for years to come as we implement the plan and use the findings to develop and refine our nursing education programs.

REFERENCES

Guba, E. G., & Lincoln, Y. S. (1989). *Fourth generation evaluation.* Newbury Park: Sage.

Popham, W. J., (Ed.) (1974). *Evaluation in education: Current applications.* Berkeley: McCutchan.

Provus, M. (1971). *Discrepancy evaluation for educational program improvement and assessment.* Berkeley: McCutchan.

Rossi, P. H., & Freeman, H. E. (1989). *Evaluation a systematic approach* (4th ed.). Newbury Park, CA: Sage.

Roth, R. A. (1978). *Handbook for evaluation of academic programs.* Washington, DC: University Press of America.

Shadish, W. R., Cook, T. D., & Leviton, L. C. (1991). *Foundations of program evaluation.* Newbury Park, CA: Sage.

Stake, R. E. (1967). The countenance of educational evaluation. *Teachers College Record, 68,* 523–540.

Stufflebeam, D. C., Foley, W. J., Gephart, W. J., Guba, E. G., Hammond, R. I., Merriman, H. O., & Provus, M. M. (1971). *Educational evaluation and decision-making.* Itasca, IL: Peacock.

Tuckman, B. W. (1979). *Evaluating instructional programs.* Boston: Allyn and Bacon.

Worthen, B. R., & Sanders, J. R. (1973). *Educational evaluation: theory and practice.* Worthington, OH: Charles A. Jones.

4

An Outcome Assessment of Liberal Education for the Baccalaureate Nursing Major

Sachiko Claus
Mary Graiver
Margaret Krawczyk
Sr. Rachel Wallace

Increasing emphasis on liberal education and the assessment of the outcomes of this component in higher education are evident in a number of reports and conference proceedings since 1980 (National Institute of Education, 1984, 1985). Professional schools, whose primary emphasis has traditionally been on the knowledge and skills in specialty areas, have recently been challenged to reconsider their educational goals (Eldman & Lynton, 1985; Coleman, 1986; Sakalys & Watson, 1985). The American Association of Colleges of Nursing (AACN) has recommended that education for the professional nurse should focus on both liberal and professional education (AACN, 1987). The Association has published an "Essential's Document" which defines college and university education for nursing.

Philosophically, baccalaureate nursing educators believe liberal or general education is essential for the graduate. Gillis (1989) proposes that general education for the professional nurse will allow the individual to reach full potential in practice, make informed ethical choices, become involved in policies for health care, and foster learning throughout the life-span.

The faculty in the department of nursing, a baccalaureate program in the university setting where this study was conducted, help shape and actively support the liberal education component of the baccalaureate nursing major. Faculty view it not only as a foundation but also as an essential part of professional nursing education. Faculty believe that learning in liberal education continues beyond the freshman and sophomore year, and that there should be continued emphasis on liberal education throughout the nursing major. The objective of this study was to measure the learning gains of the baccalaureate nursing major in the areas of liberal education competencies.

REVIEW OF LITERATURE

The literature that deals with the measurement of liberal education outcomes in nursing education has been rather sparse, in large part because of the difficulty in measuring behavioral outcomes of liberal education (Gillis, 1989). Banta (1985) reported the use of the ACT's COMP (College Outcome Measurement Project) Test, a standardized, norm-referenced test, as a valid and reliable instrument for assessing general education outcomes in various majors including nursing in the university setting. The COMP is a test of "effective adult functioning"; students are asked to apply knowledge in situations encountered in everyday living. Scores on the COMP have been shown to predict effective performance both in career and in the role of citizen.

In contrast, the following two studies have used criterion-referenced instruments that measured a set of broad, general competencies reflective of the outcomes of liberal education. DeBack and Mentkowski (1986) compared the baccalaureate nursing graduates and those from other types of nursing programs in terms of a set of broad, general competence (nursing competence). They reported that nurses with a baccalaureate degree demonstrated more nursing competencies than those from other types of nursing programs. Nursing competencies were measured through Job Competence Assessment, using a structured interview technique.

Another study conducted by Bottoms (1988) examined the relationship between competencies that are intended outcomes of liberal education as demonstrated in the behavior of nursing graduates and the type of nursing program completed by nursing graduates. Bottoms also examined the graduate's behavior, with competencies demonstrated in both personal and professional life.

The questionnaire consisted of two parts, with the first part relating to the nurses' personal lives and the last part relating to nurses' professional lives. Bottoms concluded that the outcomes of the liberal education do make a difference in the behavior of nursing graduates and that the influence of liberal education outcomes were more evident in their personal lives than in their professional lives.

BACKGROUND

Since 1985, this state-supported university, located in Michigan where this study was conducted, has participated in an "Outcome Project," as part of the dissemination phase of a nation-wide project to help campus communities develop outcome assessment through the National Center for Higher Education Management System (NCEMS). The objective of the project in the department of nursing was to measure the learning gains of the baccalaureate nursing major in the areas of liberal education competencies.

At this university, the student is selected into the college of nursing at the beginning of the second semester of the sophomore year. Prior to selection, the student is required to take liberal education courses, and prerequisite courses in physical and behavioral sciences for the nursing major. Following selection into the program, an upper division psychology course along with an upper division sociology course must be completed along with the courses in the nursing major, whose curriculum is based primarily on Roy's Adaptation model (Roy, 1984).

METHODOLOGY

A longitudinal design was used to measure the learning that has occurred within the nursing major using assessment instruments developed by the American College Testing Program (ACT) (ACT, 1985a, 1986a). These instruments, the College Outcome Measurement Project (COMP) Objective Test and the ACT Composite Examinations, identified six general outcome domains of liberal education that stress the application of knowledge in real life rather than merely recalling or engaging in mental exercises: (1) solving problems, (2) communicating, (3) functioning with social organizations, (4) using science and technologies, (5) using arts, and (6) clarifying values.

Instruments

The ACT COMP Objective test and the ACT Composite Examination, both developed and distributed by ACT (1985a, 1986a), were used as instruments to measure the outcome of liberal education.

The COMP Objective test is a paper and pencil test with a variety of activities to provide the student with an opportunity to demonstrate competence in the six areas of abilities: solving problems, communicating, functioning within social institutions, using science and technologies, using arts, and clarifying values. The instrument consists of 15 activities in which there are 60 multiple-choice questions. Several media—a newspaper clipping, a business letter, excerpts from 16 mm films, and a segment of taped music—are used as stimulus materials. The test requires two and one-half hours to administer.

A number of field tests of this instrument over the course of several years have established the validity and reliability of this test. The test-retest reliability of this instrument was reported as adequate at .78 or higher (ACT, 1981, p. 23).

The ACT Composite Examination consists of a series of 15 activities based on realistic simulations drawn from each of the six areas of abilities described above. These simulation activities require the student to apply general knowledge and skills to problems and issues commonly confronted by adults. In addition to a paper and pencil test, the Composite Examination required the student to write three short essays and to tape record three three-minute speeches according to directions provided. This examination takes four hours to complete.

The validity evidence of this instrument has been obtained from a number of studies comparing the Composite Examination subscores and job performance of various adult groups (ACT, 1981, p. 33). The alpha coefficient estimates for subtests ranged from .58 to .80. The test-retest reliability ranged between .71 and .93. The interrater agreement studied in two institutions ranged between .71 and .98. The Composite Examination is designed to measure similar types of competencies as those of the COMP Objective test. However, the ACT Composite Examination is known to provide a more indepth assessment than the ACT Comp Objective Test. The ACT recommends that since these two test results can be directly comparable, they can be used in a longitudinal study to compare scores generated by these instruments administered over time.

Subjects

All students who were admitted to the department of nursing during 1986 (winter and fall semesters, n = 44) were the subjects of this study.

Procedure

The COMP Objective test was administered as a "pre-test" measurement to all entry-level basic nursing students during the first week after they were admitted in both the winter and fall semesters of 1986 (n = 44). The students were tested in a regular classroom during one of their scheduled classes. The purpose of the project was explained to the students. The students were assured that individual results would only be available to the students themselves, that they were to be kept confidential, and that the data were to be analyzed as a group for the purpose of this study.

Each student was provided with an examination booklet, answer sheets, and number two pencils. One of the four members in the college of nursing, who were members of the outcome project, served as an examiner for each testing date. Each examiner followed the COMP Guide for Administration (ACT, 1985b) step-by-step to administer the test. A 16 mm projector, a slide projector, and an audiotape player were used for testing in addition to test booklets. The COMP Objective test took 129 minutes for both test groups to complete.

The same group of students were again tested one week prior to graduation (at the end of fall and winter classes, n = 39). The ACT Composite Examination was used for the "posttest" measurement. The student attrition in the posttest measurement resulted in a slight decrease of the sample size for this study. A videotape player and an audiotape player were used as stimulus materials. Following the paper and pencil test, each student was asked to write three short essays and also to tape record three three-minute speeches as directed in the test booklet. A language laboratory equipped with individual tape recorders and earphones was used to tape student's speeches. The entire examination lasted for four hours.

The test answer sheets, writing samples, and taped speeches collected from students were sent to the ACT for analysis after each testing. The following results and analysis were based on the report prepared by the ACT for this study.

RESULTS

A longitudinal study was conducted utilizing the results of the COMP Objective test and the ACT Composite Examination administered to the 39 students at the entry and exit levels respectively. Table 4-1 displays the mean of total test scores and subscores in each of the six areas of abilities.

Table 4-1
COMP Objective Test/Composite Examination
(OT)   (CE)
Means and Mean Gains for Nursing Program Students

	All Tested		Longitudinal Study		
	Entry (OT) 3/86-9/86 n = 44	Exit (CE) 12/88-4/88 n = 38	Entry (OT) 3/86-9/86 n = 25	Exit (CE) 4/88-2/88 n = 25	Pre/Post Gain
Total	189.5	183.2	185.2	186.6	1.4
FSI	63.2	63.0	62.4	63.9	1.5
US	64.6	61.6	63.1	63.2	0.1
UA	61.7	58.3	60.0	59.5	−0.5
COM	51.6	53.7	49.7	55.6	5.9
SP	78.0	73.2	76.6	74.4	−2.2
CV	59.5	56.1	58.6	56.8	−1.8

The mean total scores in the longitudinal study revealed a net gain of 1.4 points between the pre-tests and the posttests (from 185.2 to 186.6). Among the subscores in each of the six areas of abilities, the mean COM (communication) subscore showed a gain of 5.9, and the mean FSI (functioning in social institutions) subscore showed a gain of 1.5. The mean subscores in other areas, UA (using arts), SP (solving problems), CV (clarifying values), showed gain scores ranging from −.5 to −2.2. The mean subscore of US (using science) showed a gain of .1. Table 4-2 displays pre- and posttest mean scores plotted on reference group norms for seniors throughout the country. Overall growth for this sample as indicated by mean total score was approximately at the 44 percentile.

The evaluation and scoring of open-ended responses, essays, and short speeches were conducted by the trained staff of the ACT. The mean total speaking score at the senior level for this group was at the 68 percentile compared to the reference norm of seniors participating in the COMP tests at other four year institutions. The mean total writing score was at the 62nd percentile.

ANALYSIS AND CONCLUSIONS

A measurement of growth from entry to exit has been based on 25 usable test scores from the 39 participants. There were 13 students who demonstrated losses of 10-33 points from entry to exit. Analyses of a number of longitudinal

Table 4-2
COMP Objective Test Sample Mean
plotted on 1988 norms for seniors at selective institutions
(n = 25)

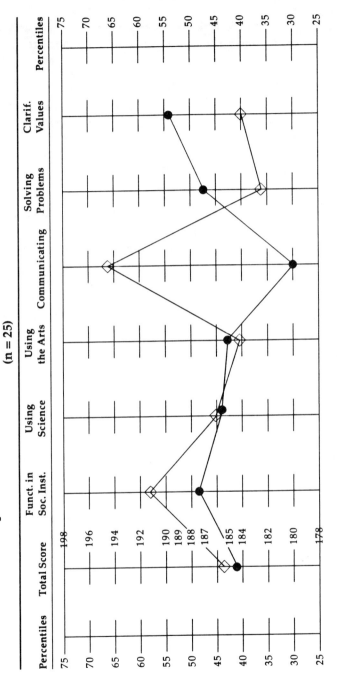

◇ = The percentile of post-test means for exiting nursing students tested 1988
● = The percentile of pre-test means for entering nursing students tested 1986

studies have indicated that losses of this magnitude raise the question of validity of the posttest score. These students were then excluded from the analysis. The estimated mean gain score of 1.4 raw score points for this group is rather small compared to the national norm, although an increase in sub-scores has been observed in some areas. The gain shown under the mean subscores in COM and FSI for this sample probably reflects the emphasis the nursing faculty placed in their teaching. Net gains in writing and speaking abilities reflected in their writing and speech sample also seem to indicate the emphasis in the curriculum. On the other hand, the negative net gains shown in SP and CV are of concern.

The small mean total gain score and negative gain scores noted in some areas of abilities might be interpreted as follows. First, the small sample size precluded meaningful comparison between the mean scores of pre- and post-tests. Second, the entering level of achievement of this sample and the refer-ence norm group were not directly comparable due to too few SAT or ACT scores available to warrant meaningful judgment about comparability. Third, the students may not have been motivated to put their best effort to achieve in this test. The conditions under which the posttests were administered may not have been the best of circumstances. The posttests were administered to the seniors one week prior to graduation, and it lasted for nearly four hours. Although all students in the graduating class were urged to participate, neither non-participation nor under-achievement in this test affected their academic records. Thus, this may have caused some students to be less moti-vated to achieve in this examination. Fourth, generalizability of this sample to the total student group of this nursing program is in question. This is due to the variability of incoming students' academic abilities above the minimum admission requirements from year-to-year and major curriculum revisions which the university has undergone since this study was conducted.

In the 1980s, outcome assessments in higher education generally took the form of the "value-added" outcome assessment method using the norm-referenced tests. The assessment data were used primarily for political and financial purposes for the educational institutions. The recent literature, how-ever, proposes the development of assessment techniques that are formative and more tailored to the academic objectives defined by each program and institution. Consequently, the assessment activities are now tied more to the improvement of academic programs and student learning (Neuman, 1990).

The experience of participating in an outcome project has provided the faculty with a great deal of insight which will help toward future efforts in the outcome assessment of student achievements. Appropriate research designs, instruments, and assessment methods of outcomes for the nursing major must be explored further.

REFERENCES

American Association of College of Nursing. (1987). *Essentials of college outcomes.* Washington, DC: The Association.

American College Testing Program. (1981). *COMP technical report.* Iowa City, IA: The ACT.

American College Testing Program. (1985a). *COMP objective test* (Form VII). Iowa City, IA: The ACT.

American College Testing Program. (1985b). *College outcome testing program: Guide for administration.* Iowa City, IA: The ACT.

American College Testing Program. (1986a). *ACT composite examination* (Form IX). Iowa City, IA: The ACT.

American College Testing Program. (1986b). *The college outcome measurement program: Guide for administration.* Iowa City, IA: The ACT.

Banta, T. (1985, October 14). *Experience with the COMP exam at the University of Tennessee, Knoxville, 1980-1985.* A paper presented at the National Conference on Assessment in Higher Education.

Bottoms, M. S. (1988). Competencies of liberal education and registered nurses' behavior. *Journal of Nursing Education, 27,* 124-130.

DeBack, V., & Mentkowski, M. (1986). Does the baccalaureate make a difference?: Differentiating nurse performance by education and experience. *Journal of Nursing Education, 25,* 275-285.

Coleman, E. (1986). On redefining the baccalaureate degree. *Nursing and Health Care, 7,* 193-196.

Eldman, S. E., & Lynton, E. A. (1985, October 13-15). *Assessment in professional education.* A paper presented at the National Conference on Assessment in Higher Education, University of South Carolina.

Gillis, A. (1989). Beyond the rhetoric: Benefits of a baccalaureate education for nursing. *Canadian Journal of Nursing Administration,* Nov/Dec, 5-8.

National Institute of Education. (1984). *Involvement in learning: Realizing the potential of American higher education.* A report of the study group on the conditions of excellence in American higher education. Kenneth P. Mortier, Chair. Washington, DC: U.S. Department of Education.

National Institute of Education. (1984, October 13-15). *The national conference on assessment in higher education.* Columbia, South Carolina.

Neuman, B. (1990). NACADA Conference, Fall, 1990. Unpublished document.

Roy, C. (1984). *Introduction to nursing: An adaptation model* (2nd ed.). Englewood Cliffs, NJ: Prentice Hall.

Sakalys, J., & Watson, J. (1985, September-October). New directions in higher education: A review of trends. *Journal of Professional Nursing,* 293-299.

5

Assessment of Affective Outcomes in RN/BSN Programs: Advancing Toward Professionalism

Ellen A. Woodman
Linda Knecht
Mary E. Periard
Eunice A. Bell

Bachelor of science in nursing (BSN) Programs are designed to develop the critical thinking skills and leadership and management capabilities needed for a professional orientation in nursing. Some students enter BSN programs as registered nurses (RN) having already completed their basic nursing education at the diploma or associate degree level. Students make the transition from the predominantly technically focused role acquired in diploma and associate degree programs to a more professionally oriented role in the baccalaureate program with varying degrees of success and at different rates.

The purpose of this study was to identify affective factors which potentially impact the RN student's transition from a technical to a professional role which encompasses a sense of autonomy, a holistic approach, the use of an extended base of knowledge, and identification with nursing as an organized profession.

RESEARCH QUESTIONS

The following research questions were addressed in this study:

1. Does the student's degree of professionalism change over the span of the program?

2. What are the relationships among selected personal, situational and motivational factors, and the professionalism of RN/BSN students?

3. Which variables are the strongest predictors of professionalism in RN/BSN students?

COMPONENTS OF PROFESSIONAL SOCIALIZATION

A review of the literature revealed that various components of the professional socialization of nurses have been studied. Some studies have focused on conceptual issues, such as, motivation (Carmody, 1982), students' perceptions about the professional role (Hillsmith, 1978), role orientation (Whelan, 1984), negative feelings during socialization (Owen, 1983), and assessment of the socialization process (Throwe & Fought, 1987). Other studies have analyzed issues around curriculum (Queen, 1984) and type of program (Beeman, 1988; Lynn, 1981; Thurber, 1988). Baker and Barlow (1988) described student, faculty and program characteristics that promoted success in BSN programs for RNs. Jacobsen (1983) found that completion of an RN/BSN program appeared to be associated with changes in work-related value systems. The transition from technical to professional outlook was measured by the following dimensions: autonomy, holism, identification with nursing as an organized profession, and belief in expanded forms of knowledge. Jacobsen concluded that it was less useful to examine professionalism as a global trait and more important to correlate or identify specific values which relate to the development of professionalism. The present study sought to extend Jacobsen's work by exploring the relationship between both previously studied and new factors and the development of professionalism.

The majority of the studies reviewed identified resocialization as the process necessary to achieve the desired level of professionalism. According to Woolley (1978), resocialization is the key to successful change. Styles (1978) described this process as the "development of a professional soul" (p. 29).

Shane (1980), described the difficulties encountered in the resocialization process as a crisis, and entitled it the "Returning to School Syndrome" (RTSS).

According to Shane (1983), "The Returning to School Syndrome" is composed of three stages: the honeymoon, the conflict, and the resolution. The first stage, *honeymoon*, represents the time when the student recognizes the similarities between past and present educational experiences. This stage ends when aspects of the student's self-image are called into question.

The second stage, *conflict*, includes a period of disintegration followed by reintegration. It begins with growing awareness of the difference between past and present. After years of practice, often in a leadership position, the student's perspective of nursing is challenged, as well as his or her self-image. Throughout the program, students perceive threats to their self-concept ranging from subtle cues to formal evaluations from faculties. As the conflict progresses, students challenge their basic values related to nursing. They examine differences between values presently held and those emphasized by the faculty and school.

The third stage, *resolution*, includes false acceptance, chronic conflict, or biculturalism (the integration of the school culture and the original nursing culture). Students who achieve biculturalism do not abandon old values, but integrate new values, understanding the significance in each. They expand their scope of practice and envelope a broadened perspective of nursing. They are self-confident, value education intrinsically, and have a positive attitude toward growth and change.

Shane (1983) suggests three key elements that promote effective coping with RTSS and enhance resocialization: having the right attitude includes trust in oneself and nursing educators; a strong support system is essential; and academic skills are required.

The elements of trust and social support cited as enhancing professional socialization in Shane's (1983) work are part of the affective domain. Affective factors have been recently emphasized in the literature as valuable student outcomes in nursing education (American Association of Colleges of Nursing, 1988; Hart & Waltz, 1988; Waltz, 1988). Characteristics in the affective domain are plagued with measurement problems and have been accorded the least importance in the past (Hart & Waltz, 1988). Hart and Waltz report the least frequently measured student outcomes as self-concept, self-esteem, social support, moral reasoning, creativity, critical thinking, professional attitude, and ethical decision making. Several of the variables examined in this study—self-concept, social support, and professional attitudes—were among the least frequently measured student outcomes.

PERSPECTIVE TRANSFORMATION

Mezirow's (1978) theory of perspective transformation forms the theoretical base for this study. This contemporary theory appears most congruent with both the "Returning to School Syndrome" and the concept of resocialization. Mezirow proposes that individual constructions of reality are dependent on reinforcement from the sociocultural world. These constructions or "reality perspectives" can be transformed by reflecting on self-experience and creating new strategies. This transformation is a developmental process with three phases analogous to the RTSS stages. First, alienation parallels the disintegration stage in Shane's (1983) work. Second, reframing parallels the reintegration stage. Third, contractual solidarity corresponds with the biculturalism of Shane's (1983) third stage.

METHODOLOGY

The present authors used the survey research method with the objective of making explanatory assertions about a population of RN/BSN students. Factors selected for examination in this study met two criteria: variables previously researched needing replication or study in a different context and variables not previously studied or reported in the literature. Predictor variables included situational, personal, and motivational. The situational variable, social support, was defined as assistance from family, friends, peers, and employers. Personal variables studied included trust, self-concept, and intolerance of ambiguity. The motivational variable was professional goals. The criterion variable, professionalism, measured the professional socialization of RN/BSN students in the four dimensions of the professional role (autonomy, holism, identification with nursing as an organized profession, and belief in expanded forms of knowledge as) reported by Jacobsen (1983). The survey design was cross-sectional. The relationships among the predictor and criterion variables were examined at three points in the RN/BSN programs. Students enrolled in the first nursing course in these programs (at mid-point) and those approaching graduation were sampled. The mid-point was included in order to examine data relative to progress toward resocialization, particularly since this was not reported in previous studies.

Sampling

A multistage cluster sample was used. The sampling frame consisted of National League for Nursing accredited RN/BSN programs in colleges and universities in the Midwest. From this sampling frame, clusters were selected. Four clusters were used to reflect a diversity in size of student enrollment, administrative control, racial mix, instructional ratio, geographical area, tuition, and admission criteria. The second stage of the design was the selection of the samples of each cluster. The sample included urban, rural, public, and private universities in four midwest states. The average number of RN/BSN students per school was 125 with a mean of 30 graduates per year. Because RN/BSN programs usually provide for self-paced progression, courses often vary considerably in the number of students enrolled. Therefore, the ability to obtain equal sample size at each of the three data collection points was limited. In each of the clusters, a convenience sample was drawn. Each student in the sample completed a packet of self-report instruments during a designated class period. A total of 296 students participated in the study.

Instruments

Six instruments were included in the study. Professionalism, the dependent variable, was measured by the Professional Values Scale developed by Jacobsen and Sabritt (1983). Three of the independent variables were measured by standardized instruments—Trustworthiness, (Wrightsman, 1964), Intolerance of Ambiguity, (Budner, 1962), and the Tennessee Self-Concept Scale (Fitts, 1965). The remaining two scales were developed by the University of Michigan-Flint faculty. Items were derived from the literature and from professional practice. Content validity is assumed. Reliability of all instruments was .76 or higher.

RESULTS

Professionalism

To answer the first research question, do students in RN programs increase in professionalism over the span of the program, analysis of the criterion variable, professionalism, was done. Data from three stages of the program, beginning, middle, and completion were analyzed. There was a significant difference in professionalism among the stages. $(F = 5.01, df = 295, p < .01)$.

Further analysis of data at two stages (beginning and completion) revealed a significant difference in professionalism scores between the two stages $(F = 10.10, p < .0001)$.

Selected Factors and Professionalism

To examine the second research question, the relationships between personal, situational and motivational factors, and professionalism, each independent variable was correlated with the dependent variable. Two of the five independent variables, professional goals and trustworthiness, correlated positively with professionalism. One variable, intolerance of ambiguity, as expected was inversely correlated with professionalism. One subscale (the social self) of the variable self-concept was positively correlated with the dependent variable. The variables support and total self-concept were not significantly related to professionalism.

Predictors of Professionalism

To examine the final research question, the relationships among the several independent variables and the dependent variable, professionalism, multiple regression techniques were utilized. Self-concept was not found to be a significant predictor variable. Professionalism was then regressed on the variables support, professional goals, trustworthiness, and intolerance of ambiguity. The regression equation resulted in an F statistic of 20.58, $p < .0001$. The variables tested accounted for 32 percent of the variance in professionalism.

DISCUSSION

The data that revealed a significant increase in professionalism over the span of the program confirmed that the RN completion programs in this study are serving their intended purpose. Students increased their professionalism in the four dimensions: autonomy, holistic practice, identification with nursing as an organized profession, and belief in expanded forms and sources of knowledge.

The measure of professionalism was taken at three stages: the beginning, midway, and at the conclusion of the educational program. Based on the analysis of variance (across stages), the growth in professionalism was gradual rather than abrupt.

Findings support resocialization as a process. A gradual increase in professionalism scores reflects the movement toward contractual solidarity described in Mezirow's (1978) theory and the biculturalism of the third stage of the "Returning to School Syndrome" (Shane, 1983). The next stage of the study examined the relationship among selected factors and professionalism. There were significant bivariate relationships between professional goals, trustworthiness, intolerance of ambiguity, and the dependent variable, professionalism.

Motivational Variables

The strong positive relationship between professional goals and professionalism confirmed that students who value professional activities such as writing and research are more likely to believe professionals use expanded forms of knowledge. Those students who are committed to involving themselves in professional organizations are more likely to believe in nursing as an organized profession. Furthermore, those students who plan involvement in community service value practice in a holistic manner.

Personal Variables

Trustworthiness was defined by Wrightsman (cited in Robinson & Shaver, 1973) as "the extent to which people are seen as moral, honest and reliable." The positive correlation between trustworthiness and professionalism reflects the ability of a professional to commit to another, that is, to trust. Successful health care delivery requires an intensely collaborative working arrangement among nurses, physicians, and other health care professionals. Furthermore, the successful delegation of components of patient care for which one is ultimately responsible depends on the willingness to trust others. Students surveyed in this study had developed the willingness to trust others. One aspect of professionalism which was not positively correlated with trustworthiness was autonomy. As scores in autonomous behaviors increased, a significant change in levels of trustworthiness did not appear. Although higher levels of autonomy may indicate a move toward more independent actions and commitment to self, it is not associated with a change in trust.

Ambiguity is defined as a state of being unsure or uncertain when facing situations which are unclear or nebulous (Budner, 1962). In the day-to-day operation of health care delivery, nurses frequently encounter situations without precise practice guidelines. Analysis of intolerance of ambiguity revealed an inverse relationship between intolerance of ambiguity and professionalism. As intolerance to ambiguity decreased, professionalism increased. This suggests that as students are better able to deal with ambiguity, their degree of professionalism increases.

Self-concept was measured with a scale comprised of five subscales: the physical, ethical-moral, personal, family, and social (Fitts, 1965). One subscale, social, was correlated positively with professionalism. The social self is identified by Fitts as the aspect of the self-concept centered on the individual's relationships with people in general. This finding suggests that nursing students who establish positive relationships with clients tend to display professional attributes.

Situational Variable

Although the data revealed a generally high level of social support from all sources, there was not a significant relationship between support and professionalism. One possible explanation for this might be that although social support is important (students often comment that it is crucial) in completing the nursing program, it was not found to impact the degree of professionalism.

CONCLUSION

Overall, students demonstrated advancement toward professionalism in RN/BSN programs. Analysis revealed that significant increases in the four dimensions of professionalism occurred over the span of the program. The study participants increased their professionalism score and passed through Mezirow's (1978) developmental stages to the point of contractual solidarity. Furthermore, the participants mastered the "Returning to School Syndrome" (Shane, 1980) and reached the final stage, biculturalism.

Exploration of two of Shane's (1983) key elements of the RTSS—support and trust—revealed mixed results. Trustworthiness was a strong predictor of professionalism in the sample studied. Support, however, was only minimally significant. The inference could be made that social support is not an absolute necessity in achieving professionalism. Those with limited support can become resocialized and develop as a professional. This finding is especially noteworthy in the current social environment. Potential nursing professionals are drawn from a population which includes many persons with limited resources. Many RN/BSN students enter programs with a great determination to achieve and few personal resources. The question arises "how to help them achieve?" One answer is found in the data from a new variable introduced in this study.

This variable, professional goals, exhibited a strong positive correlation with professionalism. It was the strongest predictor of professionalism. Thus, students who are strongly focused on professional goals appear to have the best potential for resocialization. Those who enter because they perceive it is required of them generally frame goals around "getting a piece of paper." For these students the resocialization process may be difficult and the outcome of increased professionalism limited. Students lacking professional goals should be counseled prior to admission to the BSN program. These students need to be assisted in clarifying and articulating their purposes for desiring a BSN degree and their understanding of the attributes of the professional role. Perhaps some of these potential students should be directed to other career/ educational opportunities.

Intolerance to ambiguity also was correlated with professionalism in an inverse relationship. This finding supports observations by educators that students unable to deal with ambiguity struggle with problem solving and critical thinking in complex decision making. The ability to make decisions and choose a course of action in unplanned and complex situations is critical in today's and for the future health care delivery system. Hart and Waltz (1988) note that the demands on nurses today require a "more comprehensive and complex level of nursing practice" (p. 1). It appears that the ability to tolerate ambiguous situations is a valuable characteristic of professional nurses. Further examination of this variable in professional nursing students is needed.

In summary, trustworthiness, ability to tolerate ambiguity, and having professional goals were variables associated with professionalism. It is appropriate to assess for these characteristics in RN/BSN students on admission and to support their further development throughout the program. In addition, throughout the RN/BSN program, all students should be the recipients of ongoing efforts by faculty to define, explain, and model the attributes of professionalism expected of students in the program. Faculty promotion of the value of research, publication, community service, and of student involvement in these areas enhance the development of professionalism. In addition to course work and other curricular approaches, exposure to a myriad of professionals in formal and informal settings, to research conferences, and to special symposia should be increased. The experiential approach as well as formal education programming can and should be combined to optimize students passage to the final outcome—resocialization to the professional role.

In this study, selected variables within the affective domain were examined as they relate to professionalism. Additional work—examining characteristics within the affective domain as program outcomes—is needed and supported as essential in professional nursing education by the American Association of Colleges of Nursing (1988) and by the National League for Nursing (Hart & Waltz, 1988). Now that the important elements of nursing program outcomes are being identified (Hart & Waltz, 1988), the next challenge is the development of reliable and valid measurement tools. Nursing educators and researchers need to join together as they work toward the goal of instrument development.

With appropriate tools to measure characteristics within the affective domain, research needs to continue and expand to examine the extent of these variables in students at admission to nursing programs, their relationship to professional development, and as program outcomes. Variables within the affective domain need to be integrated into ongoing program evaluation as a measure of professional nursing program quality and effectiveness.

REFERENCES

American Association of Colleges of Nursing. (1988). *Essentials of college and university education for professional nursing.* Washington, DC: Author.

Baker, S. S., & Barlow, D. J. (1988). Successful registered nurse education: A case analysis. *Nurse Educator, 13*(1), 18–22.

Beeman, P. (1988). RN's perceptions of their baccalaureate programs: Meeting their adult learning needs. *Journal of Nursing Education, 27,* 364–370.

Budner, S. (1962). Intolerance of ambiguity as a personality variable. *Journal of Personality, 30,* 29–50.

Carmody, C. (1982). Motivational orientations of registered nurse baccalaureate students. (Doctoral Dissertation, Teachers College, Columbia University, 1982). *Dissertation Abstracts International, 70,* 50055.

Fitts, W. H. (1965). *Manual: Tennessee self concept scale.* Nashville, TN: Counselor Recordings and Tests.

Fitts, W. H., Adams, J. L., Radford, G., Richard, W. C., Thomas, B. K., Thomas, M. M., & Thompson, W. (1971). *The self concept and self actualization.* (Research monograph No. 3). Nashville, TN: Counselor Recordings and Tests.

Hart, S. E., & Waltz, C. F. (Eds.). (1988). *Educational outcomes: Assessment of quality—State of the art and future directions.* New York: National League for Nursing.

Hillsmith, K. E. (1978). From RN to BSN: Student perceptions. *Nursing Outlook, 26,* 98–102.

Jacobsen, M. (1983). RN baccalaureate education: A process-product evaluation. Lexington: University of Kentucky, College of Nursing.

Lynn, M. (April, 1981). The professional socialization of nursing student: A comparison based on type of educational program. Paper presented at the Annual Meeting of the American Educational Research Association, Los Angeles, CA.

Mezirow, J. (1978). Perspective transformation. Adult Education, 28, 100–110.

Nunnally, J. C. (1978). Psychometric theory. (2nd ed.). New York: McGraw-Hill.

Owen, L. (1983). Identification of factors associated with negative feelings registered nurses experience during a resocialization procession baccalaureate nursing education. (Doctoral dissertation, Kent State University, 1983). Dissertation Abstracts International, 8400976.

Queen, P. S. (1984). Resocializing the degree-seeking RN: A curriculum thread. Journal of Nursing Education, 23, 351–353.

Robinson, J., & Shaver, P. (1973). Measures of social psychological attitudes. (rev. ed.). Ann Arbor, MI; Survey Research Center, Institute for Social Research.

Shane, D. (1980). Returning-to-school syndrome. Nursing 80, 10(6), 86–88.

Shane, D. (1983). Returning to school: A guide for nurses. Englewood Cliffs, NJ: Prentice Hall.

Styles, M. M. (1978). Why publish? Image, 10(2), 29.

Throwe, A. N., & Fought, S. G. (1987). Landmarks in the socialization process from RN to BSN. Nurse Educator, 12(6), 15–18.

Thurber, F. W. (1988). A comparison of RN students in two types of baccalaureate completion programs. Journal of Nursing Education, 27, 266–273.

Waltz, C. F. (1988). Educational outcomes: Assessment of quality—A prototype for students outcome measurement in nursing programs. New York: National League for Nursing.

Whelan, E. G. (1984). Role-orientation change among RN's in an upper division level baccalaureate program. Journal of Nursing Education, 23, 151–155.

Woolley, A. S. (1978). From RN to BSN: Faculty perception. Nursing Outlook, 26, 103–108.

Wrightsman, L. (1964). Measurement of philosophies of human nature. Psychological Reports, 14, 743–751.

6

Validation Testing: Implications for RN/BSN Curriculum Development

Sandra K. Krafft
Betty J. Caffo

Discussed here is our study pertaining to validation testing of registered nurse students, identification of some issues that emanated from it, and encouragement for dialogue and debate among educators about the curricular concerns identified.

PROBLEM

Although an empirical, rational basis for decision making is expected and supported in nursing, in the area of curriculum development, educators often make decisions by intuition, educational stereotypes, economics, or standards required by accreditation bodies. When determining curriculum needs of registered nurse students, educators have a unique challenge. These students are first educated and socialized at the associate degree or diploma level, gain experience, frequently of many years, in the practice setting, and often take on leadership roles. They then return to college to obtain a baccalaureate degree and hopefully gain increased knowledge, skills, professional identity, and career opportunities.

Even those individuals who support the traditional baccalaureate degree as the essential route to professional nursing acknowledge that some baccalaureate competencies are achieved by RNs upon admission to the upper division level. Interestingly and perhaps ironically, even this perspective seems a result of philosophical and anecdotal evidence rather than empirical support. Relative to the development of an educationally sound, nonrepetitive, purposeful course of study for RN students, educators have not thoroughly evaluated the following factors:

1. Where the gaps in essential knowledge are.
2. What content areas actually need to be stressed in the RN/BSN curriculum.
3. What competencies are achieved through work experience.

These uncertainties about the abilities of entering students create confusion about expected outcomes of the baccalaureate experience.

PURPOSE

We began our study to identify the strengths or weaknesses of RN students in traditional specialty content areas: care of adult, children, maternal, and psychiatric clients. These content areas were selected for study because they are emphasized at the associate degree and diploma level, there are standardized exams to measure knowledge in these areas, and upper-division baccalaureate programs generally require verification of this content for RN students upon entry into the upper division.

The study was initiated by the pragmatic need to continue refining the program of study that will ostensibly result in RN/BSN graduates achieving outcomes that are equivalent to those of traditional baccalaureate graduates. After all, both types of graduates have the same educational credentials and level of licensure. While we plan a more detailed analysis in a future phase, data from the type of study offered here can help educators identify new possibilities related to RN curriculum development.

RESEARCH QUESTIONS

Two questions were addressed in this study:

1. Are there differences in the knowledge of designated specialty areas between entering RN students and established baccalaureate norms, as measured by the NLN Mobility Profile II?
2. Are there differences in the knowledge of designated specialty areas between RN students educated at the associate degree level and those at the diploma level, as measured by scores on the NLN Mobility Profile II?

METHODOLOGY

The study population consists of registered nurses seeking a baccalaureate degree in nursing. Usable data from 57 associate degree graduates and 40 diploma graduates formed the sample. These individuals enrolled in one RN/BSN program over a three-year period, comprising total admissions. Only first-time test results were included.

Anticipated limitations included the scope of the study. Because we sought timely guidance for curriculum direction, we used already available data negating the opportunity to factor in age, length of work experience, or years since graduation from the basic nursing program. Second, our analysis is restricted to students from one program. It should be noted, however, that we are focusing on *entering* students and, as such, this sample reflects basic nursing programs from a number of states across the country as well as a variety of diploma and associate degree programs.

THE INSTRUMENT

The standardized examination, the National League for Nursing (NLN) Mobility Profile II, has been utilized in this RN/BSN program to validate prior nursing education for both associate degree and diploma graduates. Introduced in 1983 by the NLN, this instrument has gained wide acceptance and is designed to facilitate educational mobility. Its purpose is to evaluate previously acquired knowledge in order to assign credit and/or establish placement. The Mobility Profile II tests knowledge in four areas:

Care of the Client with a Mental Disorder

Care of the Adult Client

Care of the Child

Care of the Client during Childbearing

In establishing the baccalaureate normative group, 18-24 programs from 13-19 states participated in the four separate examination components. Students who completed each component to establish the norms ranged from 381-449. Baccalaureate students who formed the normative group were administered the test component as they neared completion of the course most related in content to the profile component.

Published validity information indicates that the tool is a content valid measurement, and questions are generally at the application level. Validity may be compromised by incongruent use of the test results. For example, if a school permits a particular course to be challenged as a result of successful completion of the Mobility Profile II, educators would need to closely inspect and compare course and profile content. Curricula with integrated content would naturally be least able to use the profile as a challenge option. Reliability has been addressed and appears sound in terms of internal consistency with coefficients ranging from .73 to .86 for the separate components.

Test results are analyzed with percentile scores which also are converted to standard scores called *decision scores*. The standardized mean for the norm group is 100, and the standard deviation is 20. In a survey conducted by Rubens (1986), it was noted that students from the normative group who generally earn grades of "C" typically achieved decision scores between 85 and 90. Subscores are provided as a part of the analysis of test results and give feedback for each student according to specific objectives and nursing process.

DATA RESULTS

To answer the research questions of group comparisons, t-tests for independent sample differences were calculated, using standardized decision scores provided with test analyses.

Results indicated that RN students as a whole achieved significantly higher scores in all areas than the normative group. Table 6-1 illustrates that group differences were dramatic for all four test components, ($p < 0.001$). As noted

Table 6-1
Comparison of RN Students
with the Normative Group

Content	RN Students Mean	SD	Norm Mean	SD	t
Mental	115.4	16.3	100	20	*9.27
Adult	124.6	12.4	100	20	*19.45
Child	116.4	13.0	100	20	*12.32
Childbearing	116.2	16.5	100	20	*9.49

*$p < 0.001$

Table 6-2
Comparison of ADN Graduates
with the Normative Group

Content	ADN Mean	SD	Norm Mean	SD	t
Mental	115.49	15.0	100	20	*7.79
Adult	122.16	10.8	100	20	*15.2
Child	113.18	11.1	100	20	*8.77
Childbearing	111.54	15.4	100	20	*5.49

*$p < 0.001$

Table 6-3
Comparison of Diploma Graduates
with the Normative Group

Content	Diploma Mean	SD	Norm Mean	SD	t
Mental	115.25	18.3	100	20	*5.27
Adult	128.07	13.6	100	20	*12.9
Child	120.87	14.1	100	20	*9.34
Childbearing	122.69	15.8	100	20	*8.96

*$p < 0.001$

Table 6–4
Comparison of Scores for
ADN and Diploma Graduates

Content	ADN Mean	Diploma Mean	t	p
Mental	115.49	115.25	0.07	0.94
Adult	122.16	128.07	−2.35	0.02
Child	113.18	120.87	−2.96	0.004
Childbearing	111.54	122.69	−3.40	0.001

in the table, registered nurse students scored highest in the examination pertaining to the adult client, with a mean standard (decision) score of 124.6 and standard deviation of 12.4. Their lowest score was in care of the client with a mental disorder, with a mean of 115.4 and standard deviation of 16.3.

Scores were then isolated for each educational level because associate degree and diploma graduates are often perceived as having different needs and competencies. Tables 6–2 and 6–3 illustrate how each subgroup compared with baccalaureate norms.

Associate degree graduates' scores on all components were significantly higher than the norm group. This group performed best on the adult component, while performance on the childbearing component was lowest and resulted in the largest variance in scores. Table 6–3 indicates that the diploma students also were significantly above the norm group on all components. Their performance was best on the adult test and lowest on the test for care of clients with mental disorders. Table 6–4 depicts the analysis of scores comparing performance of diploma and associate degree graduates. For care of the client with a mental disorder, the associate degree mean score was slightly higher, although not significantly so. In all other areas, diploma graduates scored higher.

DISCUSSION

In interpreting study results, it is noted that RN students in this sample were clearly not deficient in the specialty areas when compared to baccalaureate norms and are therefore entering with foundational knowledge in each of these areas. It also is apparent that diploma graduates demonstrated knowledge acquisition at or above that of associate degree graduates, indicating knowledge equivalent with that of associate degree graduates who had earned college credit in nursing courses. The results also are compatible with the performance of the three groups on the NCLEX licensure examination.

It is remarkable that after years of work experience, RN students achieve scores at such high levels in all specialty areas. Possible explanations may include the following:

1. A sounder foundation is created at the associate degree and diploma levels than the educational stereotype of a technical nursing education assumes.

2. Experience in the clinical area helps nurses to generalize problem-solving abilities into many specific nursing situations.

IDEAS FOR FURTHER STUDY

Future studies might include replication with data from several programs, as well as a more detailed analysis that would include analysis of subscores included with test results. This information would provide educators with a more reliable and precise assessment of strengths or weaknesses, especially in terms of nursing process.

ISSUES

Several seemingly distinct issues and questions arising from the study results pose challenges for curriculum development. The first of these issues addresses educators' concerns regarding content to be included in the baccalaureate curriculum for RN students. If we determine that registered nurse students have an existing knowledge base in the basic specialty areas, that is, care of adults, children, maternal, and psychiatric clients, what then should be the primary areas of curriculum emphasis for these individuals? Should it simply be the addition of content in community health, research, and leadership to maximize opportunities for education mobility in a timely fashion? If so, can we then say that this education indeed is similar in breadth and depth to most baccalaureate nursing programs?

Or should the demonstrated competency in the common specialty areas instead serve as a foundation for more expanded nursing content in the upper division, consisting of the addition of content in the following areas: nursing economics, nursing ethics, transcultural dimensions, advanced health assessment, complex care issues, technological dimensions of nursing, or specialty preparation. However, if topics such as these are included, we perhaps risk creating yet another new standard of preparation that falls somewhere between generic baccalaureate and graduate education. Indeed, could today's increasing numbers of baccalaureate programs that are designed exclusively for the registered nurse be fostering the establishment of new standards for baccalaureate nursing education?

A second curriculum issue confronting educators today is the need to promote a balanced curriculum while recognizing credit for earlier educational achievements. The American Association of Colleges of Nursing (1986) recommended a baccalaureate curriculum that carefully balances liberal arts, sciences, and nursing. A factor that impacts negatively on this balance is the present accreditation criterion requiring the majority of nursing credits to be earned at the upper division level. In order to comply with this criterion, educators in RN programs often reduce the transfer of previously earned nursing credits. Alternatively, a curriculum is implemented which has a disproportionate total number of nursing credits, resulting in an imbalance between nursing and the liberal arts and sciences. When a question was raised concerning this dilemma at a recent forum for revision of accreditation criteria, a response was offered that baccalaureate nursing should be similar to other collegiate programs in which the major is concentrated in the junior and senior years. This reasoning, however, does not account for the fact that, unlike most other disciplines, the majority of nurses first earn an associate degree or diploma in nursing. In fact, about 30 actual credits of nursing are included in the first two years of study. However, Caffo and Krafft (1990) found no consistency in the number of lower division nursing credits awarded RNs upon admission into programs enrolling only RN students. The range reported was 15–36 credits. This lack of uniformity in dealing with the RN student also is apparent in generic baccalaureate programs.

To adhere to the NLN (1985) position statement on awarding credit for nursing knowledge, nursing programs are effecting a wide variety of admission and placement procedures which includes validation or verification of previously learned nursing knowledge. Many baccalaureate educators continue to struggle with the "academic justness" of this practice. These same programs are free to accept transfer credits in English, anatomy, chemistry, psychology, and so on, but must "validate" nursing. We ask simply whether it is time to re-evaluate this practice as nursing education enters a new age with major changes in accreditation criteria and process? One viable option may be to use success on the NCLEX exam to assign credit for basic nursing as RNs enroll in baccalaureate programs. Does nursing have the courage to acknowledge that

associate degree and diploma graduates, by virtue of successful outcome performance on the NCLEX examination, deserve to have the hoops removed?

A fair and educationally sound approach in curriculum planning might be
to recognize that the associate degree graduate has completed a quality program in an institution of higher education with a collegiate program of study
consisting of at least 60 credits, with a minimum of 30 in nursing. Furthermore, because the diploma graduate also has consistently reflected a sound
foundation in basic nursing, should we not use the successful performance of
these individuals on the NCLEX examination to assign similar credit for basic
nursing?

There also is a growing interest within the nursing community and perhaps
most among baccalaureate advocates for the establishment of a second level of
registered nurse licensure. It is generally hoped the additional education of
baccalaureate graduates would then be reflected both in the credential issued
and in potential earning power. It is our responsibility as educators to develop
curricula that clearly facilitate the achievement of different nursing outcomes
for baccalaureate graduates. To date, has this really been accomplished for the
world to see?

Alternatives to the current educational models need to differentiate clearly
between the two levels of registered nurse practice. The following models
might be considered:

1. A two-step process similar in approach to the current associate
   degree and RN-only programs for everyone entering nursing
   education.

2. The scope of practice could be modified for associate degree graduates, with a focus on adult acute care and long-term care exclusively.
   Additional specialty content could then be included at the baccalaureate level. As the knowledge required continues to grow by leaps
   and bounds, it becomes increasingly difficult for associate degree
   educators to "cover it all" in two short years.

3. New alternatives to our existing educational models may have to be
   reviewed. "In nursing, as in all the healing professions, we do the
   routine things day after day, but once in a while we're asked to make
   a choice, to take a risk—and we do" (Sheard, 1990).

It is evident that clear differentiation in outcome performance between the
two levels of registered nurse graduates is needed on a national basis. Only
when this differentiation has been accomplished will we be able to provide
our colleagues in nursing service with the documentation needed to support
efforts to recognize and reward baccalaureate graduates.

REFERENCES

American Association of Colleges of Nursing. (1986). Essentials of college and university education for professional nursing. Washington, DC: Author.

Caffo, B., & Krafft, S. (1990). A survey of credit allocation for prior nursing education in BSN for RN programs. In C. Little (Ed.), Nursing & health care: The supplement (pp. 37–39). New York: National League for Nursing.

National League for Nursing. (1983). Criteria for the evaluation of baccalaureate and higher degree programs in nursing (5th ed.). New York: National League for Nursing.

National League for Nursing. (1985). Position statement of awarding credit for previous nursing knowledge and competency. New York: National League for Nursing.

Rubens, Y. (1986). Nursing Mobility Profile II: Report of 1986 survey. New York: National League for Nursing.

Sheard, T. (1990). 1991 Vital signs calendar. Menlo Park, CA: Addison-Wesley.

7

Developmental Programs and Remediation Strategies in Schools of Nursing

Evelyn Dupree Guice
Doris C. Ford

The academically at-risk population among students has significantly increased in many universities and colleges as students from diverse cultural and educational backgrounds are recruited and mainstreamed into the system. The presence of these students has created concern among administrators and faculty worried about attrition rates and the ability of their institutions to meet student needs. Because the instructional process may be a major factor in students' successful completion of a program of study, there is a need for effective developmental programs and remediation strategies to meet the needs of academically at-risk students.

A review of the literature suggests that most schools, perhaps all schools, whether we wish to admit this or not, have their share of academically at-risk students. These students have been categorized by a variety of terms: *disadvantaged, nontraditional, unprepared, uneducated, special, underachievers, poor test takers, minority, non-motivated, highly stressed, culturally diverse,* and so on

The authors would like to acknowledge the following faculty for their participation in this study: Dr. Portia Foster, Dr. Beth Hembree, Dr. Gail Camp, and Mrs. Paula Davis.

(Reed & Hudepohl, 1983). Regardless of the descriptive term used, the at-risk student is one whose underachievement is caused by phenomena which hamper the student's ability to learn and achieve in a course of study. The phenomena may be long term, such as academic preparation, or short term, such as illness or financial problems. However these phenomena may be overcome with student participation in faculty-planned developmental programs using various remediation strategies.

Contemporary students are no longer 20-year-olds who enrolled in college directly from high school. Many students are older, female parents who hold jobs, are from disadvantaged backgrounds, are educationally disadvantaged, are from rural areas, are from racial minority groups, are frequently foreign born with English as a second language, and the first in their family to attend college (Pinter, 1983; Wolahan & Wieczorek, 1991).

The most obvious characteristic reported that places the student at-risk is inadequate basic skills such as reading and comprehension (Ferguson, 1979; Huhn, 1976; Pinter, 1983). For example, a student may be reading at or below the 10th grade level and be expected to read and comprehend a nursing text written at the 12th grade or college level (Burris, 1987). Study skills are another basic inadequacy of the at-risk student (Allen, Nunley, & Scott-Warner, 1988; Crawford Olinger, 1988; Pinter, 1983; Rubin & Cohen, 1974). At-risk students need help with note taking, test taking, and time management (Pinter, 1983). Skillful time management is important if a student is to successfully schedule study time as well as job and family responsibilities. Also, failure to understand the financial assistance system may prevent a student from receiving financial awards which would allow reduced work loads (Pinter, 1983).

In addition to poor reading and study skills, many students have little background in math and the sciences. The older student may not only have forgotten but may be a victim of the tremendous knowledge explosion and must not only renew skills but also catch up on new developments (Pinter, 1983). Perhaps more important than overcoming the fear and anxiety of renewing and relearning skills or remembering facts is the degree of reasoning required for success in math and science. In other words, the student may not be functioning at the cognitive level his or her work demands. However, research during the last decade supports the idea that delayed cognitive development is a second, less overt characteristic of failing students.

A third characteristic frequently observed in the at-risk student is an inability to deal with affective problems (Pinter, 1983). In addition to the fear and anxiety experienced by students, some investigators (Malarkey, 1979; Smith, 1968) have reported a high dependency need among student nurses. This need may be heightened among older women who have assumed a secondary role in their household. It may be difficult for such students to assume the role of independent thinker.

In addition to these three characteristics observed in many at-risk students, there are students who choose not to achieve by the way they use time (relaxing, watching television, and fantasizing). According to Pinter (1983), relaxed admission policies in universities and colleges have resulted in the enrollment of these students who are underachievers. Patterns observed in these students are not easily altered and may require in-depth counseling and opportunities to achieve.

It is reported that many schools across the country have put mechanisms in place to enhance the at-risk student's opportunities for success. Others use various support and remediation strategies to move the student from where they are to where they want to be (Griffith & Conner, 1989; Wolahan & Wieczorek, 1991).

According to the literature, the majority of schools offer remediation in math, reading, and study skills (Rosenfeld, 1987; Rubin & Cohen, 1974). One third have remedial courses in other areas such as writing and science courses. Many schools use tutorials with faculty or peers serving as tutors (Allen, Nunley, & Scott-Warner, 1988; Burris, 1987; Hughes, 1988; Moore & Pentecost, 1979). Others report success with individual and group counseling sessions and academic advisement (Allen, Nunley, & Scott-Warner, 1988; Heins & Davis, 1972; Hughes, 1988; Moore & Pentecost, 1979). Other strategies reported include diagnostic testing such as the Nelson-Denny Reading Test, National League for Nursing (NLN) Readiness Test, and Mosby's Assess Test given initially and sequentially through the program of study (Crawford & Olinger, 1988; Wolahan & Wieczorek, 1991).

Workshops on personal skills such as time management, stress management, and study skills were reported as strategies in some schools (Crawford & Olinger, 1988; Moore & Pentecost, 1979). Others offer information on task organization, examination strategies, and memory and concentration.

Given the characteristics of the at-risk student and strategies used to meet their needs, how successful are these attempts? Two authors (Wolahan & Wieczorek, 1991) report their schools' NCLEX pass rate went from 37 percent in 1989 to 94 percent in 1990. Burris (1987) reported the NCLEX pass rate increased from 33 percent to 96 percent and student attrition rate decreased from 45 percent to 13 percent. The success rate of other programs are under study.

Two investigators (Reed & Hudepohl, 1983) have isolated characteristics of the successful program. All provided teacher/counselor interactions for the students, trained the teachers/counselors in self-concept techniques, and concerned themselves with the students' self-concept development as well as academic development.

Faculty in our College of Nursing had expressed concern over the changes observed in our student body and problems they were beginning to see emerge. Nursing faculty are faced not only with the challenge of improving the educational outcome of curriculum but with the challenge of meeting the needs of those at-risk among our student body. In an initial effort to support and assist our students and to improve our product, we designed a study to describe developmental programs and remediation strategies used in other schools of nursing throughout the state.

METHODOLOGY

A questionnaire was developed and submitted to a panel of experts to verify content validity. The proposal was submitted to the Jacksonville State University Institutional Review Board and permission was granted to conduct the study. The study was then piloted with a group of subjects and no procedural difficulties were identified.

A convenience sample (n = 31) was drawn from all schools of nursing in a southern state. The sample consisted of 9 baccalaureate, 17 associate degree, and 2 diploma. There also were three programs offering associate and baccalaureate degrees in nursing.

The questionnaire was mailed to the dean of each program with a cover letter explaining the purpose of the study and how the data would be used.

RESULTS

Data were tabulated using descriptive statistics. Over half (58%) of the schools of nursing surveyed reported no formal developmental programs for academically at-risk students.

The majority (94.7%) reported that academic advisement is a strategy used to meet students' developmental and remediation needs. Other strategies that were reported to be used included learning styles (47%), group counseling (26.3%), diagnostic testing (68.4%), tutorial programs (57.9%) and remediation programs in math, reading, and learning skills (84.2%). Stress management courses were offered in approximately half (57.9%) of the schools. Stress management strategies included time management (81.8%), peer support groups (72.7%) and group study sessions (45.4%). Many of the subjects (68.4%) offered NCLEX reviews.

In the schools which reported having developmental programs (42%), the implementation of that program was not, for the most part, the responsibility of one individual. Only 20 percent of respondents stated that the person responsible was nursing faculty. Those individuals (25%) were seldom housed in the school of nursing. These developmental programs were funded by university funds, student tuition, and grants.

DISCUSSION

Overall, the results suggest that structured remediation programs were not offered in the majority of schools of nursing. Strategies used to meet student developmental needs included learning styles assessment, math, reading, writing, group counseling, diagnostic testing, tutorial programs, NCLEX reviews, study skills, and stress management courses.

These findings imply that educators who are planning programs for the at-risk students should consider and include strategies to improve the student's self-concept as well as improve basic skills. As attrition rates among the at-risk population of students are reduced, there may be an increase in the number of competent graduates. This may play a role in reducing the nursing shortage as well as improving patient care. Lastly, these findings imply a need for further research of students' perceptions of their educational needs.

Based on the findings of this study, it is recommended that educators research, plan, and implement structured remediation programs in schools of nursing for academically at-risk students. It also is recommended that personnel with expertise in nursing be designated the responsibility of remediating students. In addition, further research is needed on strategies which are most effective in impacting positively on student outcomes. Last, it is recommended that this study be replicated in several different geographic locations to test situation-specificity and validity of the findings.

REFERENCES

Allen, M. E., Nunley, J. C., & Scott-Warner, M. (1988). Recruitment and retention of black students in baccalaureate nursing programs. *Journal of Nursing Education*, 27(3).

Burris, B. M. (1987). Reaching educationally disadvantaged students. *American Journal of Nursing*, 87(1), 1359–1360.

Crawford, L. A., & Olinger, B. H. (1988). Recruitment and retention of nursing students from diverse cultural backgrounds. *Journal of Nursing Education, 27*(8), 379-381.

Heins, M. J., & Davis, M. (1972). A second chance: A successful summer program prepared "high-risk" students for success in nursing school. *Hospitals,* January 72, 74-78.

Hudepohl, N. C., & Reed, S. B. (1984). High-risk students: Establishing a student retention program, part 2. *Nurse Educator, 9*(3), 19-24.

Hughes, R. B. (1988). The nursing resource center. *Journal of Professional Nursing, 4*(4), 289-293.

Moore, B. M., & Pentecost, W. L. (1979). CSULB nursing: Educationally disadvantaged students can succeed. *Journal of Nursing Education, 18,* 50-58.

Pinter, K. (1983). Support systems for health professions students. *Journal of Nursing Education, 22*(6), 232-235.

Reed, S. B., & Hudepohl, N. C. (1985). High-risk students: Evaluating a student retention program part 3. *Nurse Educator, 10*(5), 32-38.

Reed, S. B., & Hudepohl, N. C. (1983). High-risk nursing students: Emergence of remedial/developmental programs. *Nurse Educator, 8*(4), 21-26.

Rosenfeld, P. (1987). Nursing education in crisis—A look at recruitment and retention. *Nursing and Health Care, 8*(5), 283-286.

Rubin, H. S., & Cohen, H. A. (1974). Group counseling and remediation: A two-faceted intervention approach to the problem of attrition in nursing education. *Journal of Educational Research, 67*(5), 195-198.

Walker, P. (1983). The need for support services for minority pre-allied health majors. *Journal of Allied Health, 11*(1), 29-34.

Wolahan, C. G. H., & Wieczorek, R. R. (1991). Enrichment education: Key to NCLEX success. *Nursing and Health Care, 12*(5), 234-239.

8

The Measurement Characteristics of Computerized Clinical Simulation Tests (CST)

Anna Bersky

WHAT IS CST?

CST is an uncued examination which permits examinees to realistically simulate the clinical decision-making skills used in the management of client needs. The National Council of State Boards of Nursing has undertaken the study of CST to evaluate its effectiveness in testing clinical decision-making competence in nursing.

THE CST PROJECT

The CST Project is a three year, $1.9 million dollar study funded by the W. K. Kellogg Foundation. The National Board of Medical Examiners (NBME) developed a computer simulation model for testing clinical decision-making competence in medicine. The National Council has worked in collaboration with NBME to adapt their simulation model to nursing.

To date, 25 cases have been programmed, 25 scoring keys have been developed, and two cases have videodisc augmentation. A 2,500 term default nursing intervention database enables CST to function as a unique uncued examination since it is programmed to recognize a full range of nursing activities specified by examinees through free keyboard entry. A small-scale field study (77 recent graduates from 10 schools of nursing) and a large-scale pilot study have been conducted to examine the feasibility, validity, and reliability of CST.

HOW CST WORKS

Since the examination is uncued by questions or response options, the examinee must pose his or her own questions and specify his or her desired actions while working through each case. At the beginning of each case, the examinee is presented with a brief description of the client situation as well as the current case day and time. The examinee then interacts with the client over time through data collection and intervention activities which are specified through free keyboard entry. As the case progresses, client condition changes both in response to nursing action and because of the underlying problem. At any point in the case, the examinee may advance the clock in simulated time in order to further evaluate the client and take additional action. As nursing actions are specified by the examinee, each action as well as its time and sequence of performance is recorded. These features enable the implementation of scoring procedures which can award credit not only for different but equally valid nursing actions, but can also award different amounts of credit depending on the timing, sequencing, and level of correctness of nursing actions.

THE CST PILOT STUDY

The CST Pilot Study was conducted December, 1990, through January, 1991, in Chicago, Philadelphia, and Indianapolis. Two hundred sixty-three NCLEX-RN licensure candidates from 24 schools of nursing representing Diploma, ADN, and BSN education programs participated in the pilot study. On the first day, candidates were given a four-hour preparation session during which they took a 40-minute CST orientation program and five practice cases. The CST examination was taken on a subsequent day, and the amount of time needed to complete the 11-case CST exam ranged from three to six hours, depending on the examinee.

Orientation sessions were facilitated by nurse educators who themselves had completed an extensive orientation to the mechanics of CST and the content of the practice cases. The facilitator assisted examinees with both the technical and content aspects of working through CST cases. The purpose of providing examinees with the orientation and practice cases facilitated by nurse educators was to reduce the impact of a "practice effect" on examinee performance. Many candidates indicated that the orientation and practice cases provided sufficient preparation, while others indicated that they would have liked to have had experience with CST during their educational program. No practice effect was detected in analysis of the data.

ANALYSIS AND RESULTS

The results of the analyses indicate that CST is a potentially reliable and valid exam and that reliable estimates of examinee ability can be obtained. Data for the 11 CST examination cases were analyzed using the Rasch Partial Credit Model (RPCM), an application of Item Response Theory (IRT). BIGSTEPS, a computer program designed to construct Rasch measurement, was used to estimate: (a) calibrations for items; (b) calibrations for the different ordered response category structures present in the CST scoring items when timing, sequencing, and/or level of correctness are taken into consideration; and, (c) measures of person ability. Internal consistency reliability coefficients (which indicate the consistency with which the items within each case measure the candidate) for each case were obtained and ranged from .69 to .87.

Intercase reliability estimates were obtained using Cronbach's Coefficient Alpha. The intercase alpha reliability coefficients ranged from 0.86 to 0.89 depending on the sequence in which the cases were administered. These findings suggest that CST has the potential to provide reliable estimates of examinee ability.

Prior to conducting the CST Pilot Study, an analysis of the CST cases and scoring keys was performed to determine which combination of CST cases would provide the highest content validity for the CST Pilot Study examination. The analysis consisted of the following: (1) analysis of case content in terms of setting, client age, and nursing diagnoses; (2) analysis of case scoring key items and assignment of each item to one of the four client need categories specified in the current NCLEX-RN Test Plan.

1. Cases included clients with an age range from neonate to 77 years and a wide variety of nursing diagnoses. Cases were representative of a outpatient, home, and long-term care settings, as well as a variety of acute care settings (neonatal, medical-surgical, psychiatric, obstetric, and pediatric units).

2. Analysis and categorization of scoring key items indicated that the composite of items across CST cases were distributed across the four client need categories specified in the NCLEX-RN Test Plan. The weighting of items in the CST examination across the four client need categories closely approximated those specified in the NCLEX-RN Test Plan.

CONCLUSIONS AND FUTURE DIRECTIONS

The results of the CST Pilot Study provide preliminary evidence that a valid and reliable CST examination can be constructed to evaluate clinical decision-making competence in nursing. Subsequent to receiving a full report of the pilot study results at the Annual Meeting of the National Council, July 30–August 2, 1991, the delegates directed that research and development of CST be continued.

PILOT STUDY PARTICIPANT REACTIONS TO CST

"It was fun. It made me think of nursing interventions, not just choosing from a multiple choice list. It made the test-taker more active in participation." (Kenneth Barachko, Our Lady of Lourdes School of Nursing, Camden, NJ.)

"It gave me an opportunity to be in a real patient care situation and allowed me to make the decisions, not just pick an answer." (Pamela Meduga, St. Xavier College, Chicago, IL.)

"I think this test assesses critical thinking skills better than multiple choice." (Mary Coers, St. Francis College, Peoria, IL.)

"It was very interesting and it really made me think and prioritize the needs of the patient." (Keith Muska, Triton College, River Grove, IL.)

"I enjoy new experiences . . . it was like being in a real situation." (Sandra Reardon, Joliet Jr. College, Joliet, IL.)

"The patient was right there expressing signs and symptoms and feelings; better performance." (Patricia O'Connor, Frankford Hospital School of Nursing, Philadelphia, PA.)

"I was able to get more involved with the clients. It felt real, I really wanted to help the patient." (Stephen Bliss, Montgomery County Community College, Bluebell, PA.)

9

Development of an Instrument to Measure Thinking, Learning, and Creativity: A Triangulation Process

Ann M. Gothler
Mary Beth Hanner

Thinking, learning, and creativity (TLC) have been identified as factors that are critical for maintaining employees in the workplace (Naisbett & Aburdene, 1985). The best and brightest employees are attracted to work environments that foster individual growth and promote TLC. In nursing, we have been confronted with a workplace which demands that the staff nurse meet client needs, but does not focus on the personal or professional development of the individual nurse. Although in our investigation of the quality of work life of the nurse it was necessary to examine TLC, there was no available instrument for that purpose.

Thriving in our information society has been the focus of a new framework for analyzing management (Naisbett & Aburdene 1985; Peters, 1987). Newer management strategies have created a decrease in middle management; the expert is encouraged to remain at the service delivery level. The emphasis on problem analysis, innovation, and quality in the workplace creates the need for workers who are expert problem solvers, consultants, and creative idea people who are focused on the delivery of service to the consumer. Naisbett and Aburdene indicate that the presence of TLC in the workplace will be essential to attract and maintain competent workers in the nineties.

The concept of TLC encompasses the ability to do problem analysis, to synthesize ideas, and to make inferences. These skills combined with openness and curiosity about new information bring about innovation and new approaches to complex issues.

The purpose of this study were to: (1) describe nurses' perceptions of their ability to think, learn, and be creative in their current workplace; (2) examine TLC in relation to the quality of the work life for registered nurses; and (3) develop an instrument to measure TLC. The questions for the study focused on the relationship between demographic characteristics of the nurse, the characteristics of the nursing position, self-esteem, thinking, learning, and creativity (TLC), collegial interaction, job satisfaction, autonomy, interaction, and the effect on the quality of work life.

REVIEW OF THE LITERATURE

While there is considerable research on stress, burnout, and satisfaction of nurses, very limited research has been done to investigate whether nurses perceive their work environment as facilitating their growth as professionals and as individuals. One study based on Naisbett and Aburdene's (1985) ideas has reported strong growth needs among a volunteer group of RNs, particularly those under 30 years of age. This study showed that nurses in staff positions showed significantly lower satisfaction ratings than other nursing positions. Selected questionnaire items were taken from the Job Diagnostic Survey (Hackman & Oldham, 1980) with six items identified as "growth need and strength." The reliability and validity of the modified instrument and the subset of items were not discussed (Harrison, 1987).

METHODOLOGY

The design for this descriptive correlational study involved using a questionnaire for data collection. As part of a cluster group project, the data collection was done by 12 graduate students in 12 sites in four states with a response from nurses in 46 agencies (23 hospitals and 23 non-hospitals) with a total of 1,950 usable responses (approximately a 50% response rate overall). There was a lower response rate for the open-ended questions with those nurses with lower TLC being less likely to fill in the open-ended questions. After these 12 studies were completed, a meta-analysis was done to analyze the aggregate data. Four additional graduate students conducted a secondary analysis of the qualitative responses.

INSTRUMENT DEVELOPMENT: TRIANGULATION

As part of the instrument development for our study the decision was made to use triangulation with a combination of measurement approaches. The term *triangulation* was used in World War II in relation to searching for a lost ship that was transmitting radio messages for help. It was necessary to have the messages received by three different receivers in order to find the ship in the ocean or to "triangulate in" on the ship.

The original concept of triangulation in measurement was developed through the work of Campbell and his associates primarily in the quantitative research area (Campbell, 1966; Campbell & Fiske, 1955; Cook & Campbell, 1979; Webb, Campbell, Schwartz, & Sechrest, 1966). The triangulation model is based on the idea that through multiple methods we can more clearly understand the construct under study, and thereby increase the validity of the measurement. Advocates of triangulation support a multioperation, multimethod paradigm with the view that the whole is greater than the sum of its parts when both qualitative and quantitative approaches are used (Smith, 1986).

Newer views of triangulation include the bracketing model which suggests that each method should be considered as an estimate of the "correct" answer and, therefore, a range of possible answers should be used to report one's conclusions. A complementary purposes model includes overlapping approaches to measuring a construct to enhance interpretability, particularly the use of narrative questions to complement the statistical results of a quantitative study (Mark & Shotland, 1987).

INSTRUMENT DEVELOPMENT

The broad concept of triangulation was used to develop an instrument to identify the effect of TLC on the perceived quality of work life and work satisfaction. Since there were no measures of TLC in the literature and it has not been defined for nursing practice, it was necessary to develop an instrument for this study. As part of the development of a valid instrument, the cluster group of graduate students met to discuss the ways that nurses think and learn in their nursing careers. Using factor analysis, the instrument was developed and refined to have a series of subscales to "triangulate in" on measuring the concept of TLC.

The TLC instrument has five components as shown in Figure 9-1:

1. Collegial interaction (Likert-type scale) on how much planned or informal discussion takes place with other nurses in eight areas such as client problems, information in nursing journals, and nursing issues (r = .82).

2. Activities important to nurse as part of work role (Likert-type scale; 14 items) such as attending staff development programs, working on committees, and teaching staff (r = .85).

3. TLC attitude was measured using a three-part semantic differential asking nurses how they felt about Thinking (r = .77), Learning (r = .88), and Creativity (r = .89) in their current position. Factor analysis was used to refine this portion with the final version for TLC having a reliability of .93.

4. TLC—Three Cantril ladders were used, one for each of the broad concepts of thinking, learning, and creativity in order to look at each individual's summary judgment vs. her response to the semantic

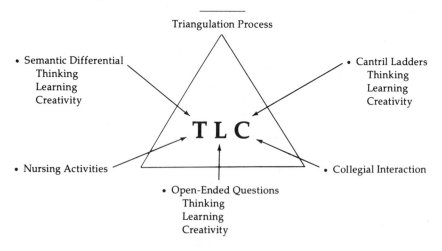

Figure 9-1
Thinking, Learning, Creativity

differential ($r = .79$ for the combination of the three items). The vertical ladder had 10 numbers from 0 to 9 with 0 identified as minimum, 4.5 as average, and 9 as maximum.

5. Open ended questions—three open ended questions asked for examples, of how the nurse was able to think, learn, and be creative in the workplace.

In addition to TLC, the study instrument contained questions about demographic information, current position, self-esteem, job satisfaction (Hinshaw, Smeltzer, & Atwood 1987), and perceptions of quality of worklife. The total six-page instrument was pilot tested and refined.

RESULTS

For the 1,950 respondents, their mean age was 37 years (range was 20 to 73 years). The mean number of years in current position was eight; mean number of years employed as a registered nurse was 12.9. Sixty-nine percent of the respondents were direct care providers. Eighty-one percent of the respondents worked in hospitals; 70 percent were employed full-time. Nurses who had a baccalaureate degree in nursing comprised 32 percent of the respondents.

In the overall study, TLC was highly correlated with and shown to be a predictor of nurse satisfaction and with perceived quality of work life. The perceived quality of work life was significantly lower for direct care providers, higher for community nurses, and higher for head nurses and clinical nurse specialists.

The TLC instrument showed that nurses in hospitals valued their interaction with physicians most highly as a source of collegial interaction. Direct care providers and nurses who were responsible for inspecting hospitals for the state had significantly lower TLC than those in other positions. Head nurses and clinical specialists had significantly higher TLC. TLC was higher for non-hospital nurses and for nurses with baccalaureate preparation. TLC was lowest for nurses whose original nursing education was at the associate degree level.

As part of the analysis, the nurses were asked how long they expected to remain in their position. The quality of work life (QWL) Cantril ladder and all the TLC measures demonstrated a consistent linear relationship. Those who expected to leave their position had the lowest QWL and TLC stepping up gradually to those who expected to stay in a position 10 years having the highest TLC and QWL (p < .0000).

ANALYSIS OF QUALITATIVE RESULTS

In the open-ended questions, nurses were asked to cite specific ways in which they were able to think, learn, and be creative in their jobs. A content analysis of the responses was done through categorization based on recognition of persistent words, phrases, themes, or concepts. Respondents were then grouped according to their responses to the Cantril ladder measure of their perceived quality of work life (QWL). High QWL was considered to be greater than six (on a 0 to 9 point scale); a low QWL score was less than four. The mid-range group was eliminated from this portion of the study.

The results of the qualitative analysis indicated that nurses with high quality of work life reported more active self-directed approaches to thinking and learning on the job. They cited direct patient care, reading articles and books, daily work experiences, and a variety of other activities in which they actively sought new knowledge. Nurses who reported low quality of work life listed more passive activities such as lectures, committee work, and clinical demonstrations as ways in which they were able to think and learn.

The question on creativity created the most difficulty and consternation for all respondents. The low QWL group often left this question blank or they wrote a negative response. The high QWL group also wrote some negative responses, although less frequently. Negative responses included such comments as: "I don't have time to be creative" and "The nature of my job prevents creativity."

Nurses with high QWL did have many positive comments as to how they were creative. Direct patient care was cited most frequently. Specific categories mentioned were: managing large groups of clients with limited resources, time management, and clinical judgment. Health teaching was frequently listed, especially in the areas of discharge planning and teaching self-care activities. One nurse stated: "I consider myself creative whenever I find innovative ways to provide cost-effective quality care."

In general, nurses in management positions cited the most opportunities to demonstrate creativity. They stated that their current management responsibilities allowed for more professional autonomy and thus they had more opportunities to be creative in their jobs. Areas frequently mentioned included developing patient care assignments, obtaining appropriate staff levels, communication, and conflict resolution.

LIMITATIONS

The study was conducted in medium and small cities and rural areas via a convenience sample; in most cases, all hospitals and other major nurse employers in an area were approached to participate in the study. There has been no investigation done in hospitals in large urban areas up to this time. Although there was remarkable consistency across the 12 regions, further investigation needs to be done to determine if there is a difference in nursing practice in large urban areas.

The length of the questionnaire at six pages with both short-answer and open-ended questions was probably a limitation. In pilot testing with graduate students, the questionnaire took about 20 minutes to complete. However, it is likely that it took the nurses a longer time to complete the questionnaire since they did not have a verbal introduction to establish the purpose of the study.

There were 12 graduate students who did the data collection for the study and another four students who analyzed the qualitative responses. Although there was extensive orientation and training for interrater reliability, and consistency in data collection and analysis, there is always a possibility for inconsistency in approach.

SIGNIFICANCE OF THE STUDY

The concept of TLC will become increasingly important in nursing and nursing education. In traditional education approaches, the learner has been the passive receiver of information; in contrast, now it is important to teach students and nurses how to think, learn, and be creative in nursing practice in order to continue their professional growth and be satisfied with their quality of work life.

The use of triangulation to develop this TLC instrument has shown that TLC is a characteristic of nursing practice that can be measured. This TLC instrument has potential for use by agencies to measure the nurses' perception of their individual growth through thinking, learning, and creativity in their work life. The instrument also can be used to evaluate the effect of organizational efforts to increase TLC in order to enhance work satisfaction and perceived quality of work life.

SUMMARY

The process of triangulation was used to develop an instrument to measure thinking, learning, and creativity in the nursing workplace. A TLC instrument consisting of five components was systematically developed as part of this study. In this descriptive correlative study, we investigated nurses' perceptions of their ability to think, learn, and be creative in their work life. The results of the investigation showed that TLC is significantly related to the perceived quality of work life of practicing registered professional nurses supporting Naisbett and Aburdene's (1985) idea that TLC is essential to attract and retain employees in the workplace.

REFERENCES

Campbell, D. T., & Fiske, D. W. (1959). Convergent and discriminant validation by the multitrait-multimethod matrix. *Psychological Bulletin, 56,* 81–105.

Campbell, D. T., & Stanley, J. C. (1966). *Experimental and quasiexperimental designs for research.* Stokie, IL: Rand McNally.

Cook, T. D. (1985). Post positivist critical multiplism. In R. L. Shotland & M. M. Mark (Eds.), *Social science and social policy.* Beverly Hills: Sage Publications.

Cook, T. D., & Reichardt, C. S. (Eds.) (1979). *Qualitative and quantitative methods in evaluation research,* Beverly Hills: Sage Publications.

Fiske, D. W. (1982). Convergent-discriminant validation in measurements and research strategies. In D. Brinberg & L. H. Kidder (Eds.), *Forms of validity in research. New directions for methodology of social and behavioral science, 12,* San Francisco: Jossey-Bass.

Hackman, J. R., & Oldhman, G. R. (1975). Development of the job diagnostic survey. *Journal of Applied Psychology, 60,* 1559–1700.

Harrison, J. K. (1987). Tuning in to the growth needs of registered nurses. *Nursing Economics 5(6),* 297–303.

Hinshaw, A., Smeltzer, C. H., Atwood, J. R. (1987). Innovative retention strategies of nursing staff. *Journal of Nursing Administration, 17(6),* 8–18.

Jick, J. D. (1983). Mixing qualitative and quantitative methods: Triangulation in action. In J. Van Maanen (Ed.), *Qualitative Methodology.* Beverly Hills: Sage Publications, 135–148.

Mark, M. M., & Shotland, R. L. (1987). Alternative models for the use of multiple methods. In M. M. Mark & R. L. Shotland (Ed.), *Multiple methods in program evaluation. New Directions for program evaluation, 35.* San Francisco: Jossey-Bass.

Mathison, S. (1988). Why triangulate? *Educational Researcher, 17*(2), 13–17.

Mitchell, E. S. (1986). Multiple triangulation: A methodology for nursing science. *Advances in nursing science, 8*(3), 18–26.

Morse, J. M. (1991, March/April). Approaches to qualitative-quantitative methodological triangulation. *Nursing Research 40*(2), 120–121.

Naisbett, J., & Aburdene, P. (1985). *Reinventing the corporation.* New York: Warner Books.

Peters, T. (1987). *Thriving on chaos: Handbook for a management revolution.* New York: Alfred A. Knopf.

Smith, M. L. (1986). The whole is greater: Combining qualitative and quantitative approaches in evaluation studies. In Williams, D. D. (Ed.), *Naturalistic evaluation. New Directions for program evaluation.* San Francisco: Jossey-Bass.

Swanson-Kauffman, K. M. (1986). A combined qualitative methodology for nursing research. *Advances in Nursing Science 8*(3), 58–69.

Webb, E. J., Campbell, D. T., Schwartz, R. D., & Sechrest, L. (1966). *Unobtrusive measures: Nonreactive research in the social sciences.* Skokie, IL: Rand McNally.

10

Curricula of Doctoral Programs in Nursing

Mary M. Ziemer
M. Louise Fitzpatrick
Theresa Valiga
Claire Manfredi
Janie Brown

INTRODUCTION

Doctoral education for nurses began in the mid 1920s in graduate schools of education (Murphy, 1981). Early programs emphasized application of educational theory and preparation for administrative roles. During the 1960s, the demand for graduates was high as baccalaureate and master's level nursing programs rapidly expanded in colleges and universities resulting in a gradual increase in the number of doctoral programs in nursing. By 1982, there were 23 programs (Murphy, 1981); currently, there are 54 programs (Sigma Theta Tau, 1991).

Doctoral programs have been independently established by participating faculty at educational institutions and, like doctoral programs in other disciplines, are regulated only by the academic institution that grants the degree. Broad parameters that reflect doctoral programs of quality have been established (American Association of Colleges of Nursing, 1987), although no previous data exist regarding the extent to which doctoral programs conform to these indicators of quality. Data collected here suggest that curricular elements in doctoral programs do not entirely meet the broad guidelines for quality suggested by the American Association of Colleges of Nursing.

HISTORICAL DEVELOPMENT OF DOCTORAL PROGRAMS IN NURSING

Development of doctoral programs in nursing has not occurred without controversy, and nurse educators have debated whether doctoral nursing education should reflect a clinical or a research orientation (Murphy, 1981). Furthermore, partly because doctoral nursing education began in graduate schools of education, questions have been raised as to the nature of the preferred degree.

Concern for the development of a research- and theory-based body of knowledge for nursing as a clinically focused discipline resulted in the development of a professional doctorate, the Doctor of Nursing Science (DNS), and increased interest in designating the traditional research degree, the Doctor of Philosophy (PhD), as the preferred credential. Initial expectations were that particular doctoral programs would reflect the emphasis appropriate to the degree awarded. The Doctor of Education (EdD) degree would emphasize role preparation for positions in educational administration, the Doctor of Nursing Science (DNS) degree would focus on clinical practice, and the Doctor of Philosophy (PhD) degree would emphasize theoretical research in the discipline.

Initially, administrative receptivity to PhD programs in nursing was lukewarm and educators could not obtain approval for new initiatives in many universities. In some cases, provision of a DNS degree program was approved as a compromise, although such programs were occasionally instituted because there was genuine belief that it was the appropriate credential for nurses whose scholarly concerns were directed to clinical practice.

To educate a critical mass of nurses with skills to conduct research and serve as faculty, the federal government funded the Nurse Scientist Program to prepare nursing candidates at the doctoral level. From 1962 to 1974, this program provided study in disciplines such as anatomy, biology, physiology, psychology, and sociology. Nurse graduates of this program who assumed academic positions were thought to be in the best position to foster development of nursing theory and research, a role which few others could fulfill.

As doctoral programs proliferated from the mid 1970s through the mid 1980s, degree-specific curricula gradually diminished, programs offering the PhD and the DNS became nearly indistinguishable (Grace, 1989; Meleis, 1988), and many programs that initially offered the DNS began to offer the PhD in nursing. Moreover, distinctions regarding the type of research that might emanate from these different types of programs were difficult to distinguish (Downs, 1989; Loomis, 1985). The organizational structure under which nursing doctoral programs existed, however, still required some programs to continue to offer degrees other than the PhD.

Periodic conferences that focused on the development of doctoral education in nursing helped to clarify priorities and create consensus about essential doctoral program components. In 1986, a position statement was endorsed by the American Association of Colleges of Nursing (AACN) and later published (AACN, 1987). This document addressed faculty quality, expectations of faculty and students, student characteristics, and the role of research in doctoral programs. Although curricular paradigms vary, common elements considered essential for all programs also were specified in broad categories. Curricular features deemed essential for a high quality doctoral program included:

1. History and philosophy and their relation to the development of nursing knowledge.
2. Existing substantive nursing knowledge.
3. Theory construction.
4. Social, ethical, and political issues of importance to the discipline.
5. Research designs, methods, and techniques of analysis appropriate to the level of doctoral study.
6. Data management, tools, and technology.
7. Student research opportunities. (AACN, 1987, p. 72)

PURPOSE

The extent to which curricula of doctoral nursing programs meet the guidelines for quality suggested by AACN has not been evaluated. Ziemer et al. (in press) have previously reported on the philosophy, degree requirements, admission requirements, and other curriculum components of doctoral education. This current analysis was undertaken to evaluate the extent to which such programs possess the elements of quality deemed essential by the AACN Position Statement (1987).

METHOD

Doctoral programs listed in *Graduate Education in Nursing* (National League for Nursing, 1988) were solicited to obtain program materials normally distributed to potential applicants. Typical information included catalogues, course requirements, and program descriptions. The nature of courses and credit requirements were identified. In some instances schools were contacted to clarify catalogue data or credit requirements when course unit allocations were listed. To enhance reliability, since the data were relatively unstructured, investigators worked in pairs to focus on particular sections of the curriculum.

RESULTS

Of the 44 schools with doctoral programs, 30 were located in public institutions, 11 were in private universities, and two were in religious institutions. Thirty-one programs offered the PhD, 11 offered the DNS, and one offered the EdD. Both the DNS and PhD were offered by one university.

Total credit requirements for completion of the doctoral degree ranged from 39 to 114. However, it was found that the standard doctoral program required completion of 60 credits, 48 in nursing, and 12 in cognate or elective courses (see Ziemer et al., in press). Programs varied considerably in the extent to which they provided the curricular elements suggested by the consensus of doctoral nurse educators as indicators of quality (AACN, 1987).

History and Philosophy and Development of Nursing Knowledge

Although "history and philosophy and their relationship to the development of nursing knowledge" was identified as one indicator of quality in a doctoral program, none of the programs studied specifically required a history or history of science component, either as a separate course or as part of a course, although 42 (95%) programs required a course in philosophy. Typically, the philosophy course was provided by the nursing department (66%), but in some programs (27%) the course was offered outside of the department. The mean number of philosophy credits required was 4.6, and the mode was 3 credits.

Existing Substantive Nursing Knowledge

In this analysis of doctoral nursing curricula, "existing substantive nursing knowledge" was defined as content and learning experiences related to the practice of nursing and the utilization of the science of nursing. Only 18 (41%) of the doctoral programs surveyed prepared clinicians and provided advanced clinical nursing courses to support this goal. Of these, 12 offered one clinical focus and six offered more than one. The clinical areas of study and the number of programs providing these clinical emphases are as follows:

Integrated Clinical Nursing (n = 12)

Psychiatric/Mental Health Nursing (n = 8)

Medical-Surgical Nursing (n = 6)

Community Health Nursing (n = 6)

Parent-Child-Family Health Nursing (n = 4)

Obstetrical Nursing (n = 2)

Gerontological Health Nursing (n = 2)

Pediatric Nursing (n = 1)

Programs which incorporated clinical nursing courses required from 3 to 24 credits in this area (approximately 12% to 20% of the total credit requirements). The mean number of credits required was 11, and the mode was 6.

Theory Construction

Curricular attention to theory construction is an essential element of doctoral curricula (AACN, 1987). Thirty-nine (89%) of the programs evaluated required course work labeled nursing theory or nursing science. The number of credits allocated to nursing theory or nursing science ranged from 3 to 15, with 6 as the modal number of credits.

Social, Ethical, and Political Issues

Twenty-six (59%) of the programs evaluated in this study included at least one 3 credit course that addressed issues in nursing; of these, 10 programs required more than 6 credits. Only one program identified a required course in health policy. The remaining 17 programs required no courses related to the "social, ethical, and policy issues of importance to the discipline" (AACN, 1987, p. 72).

Research Designs, Methods, and Techniques

The emphasis of doctoral education is on preparation for the conduct of research, and programs of quality emphasize the development of research skills (AACN, 1987). Thirty-nine of the 44 programs studied (89%) identified a generic research course provided by the nursing department as a requirement; 23 programs (52%) included research courses outside of nursing. Other course categories that focused on research skills included quantitative and qualitative analysis which were offered by 33 (75%) and 16 (36%) programs, respectively. Furthermore, research opportunities with faculty included experiences with credit allocations in 28 (67%) programs. Using modal data, up to one-half (approximately 30 credits) of all required courses in doctoral nursing programs specifically attend to the development of research skills. All schools reviewed provided emphasis on research skill development.

Data Management, Tools, and Technology

For purposes of this study, data management, tools, and technology were defined as coursework related to use of computers. Formalized computer courses were offered in only 12 (27%) of the 44 doctoral programs studied. However, descriptions of other courses included in the curriculum suggested that computer competency may be developed as part of other courses in eight additional schools. Only five programs explicitly stated that they required computer competency to complete their program. Two of these five programs, as well as three additional programs, recognized computer literacy in lieu of a foreign language required of doctoral candidates.

Student Research Opportunities

Because a major objective of doctoral study is to develop research competence, the availability of student research opportunities was expected to feature significantly in the programs analyzed. The curricula reviewed did appear to reflect this value as 28 (67%) of the programs analyzed included structured for-credit opportunities for student participation in the research process. These opportunities included collaborative work with faculty, independent study projects for academic credit, and dissertation work.

The most ubiquitous opportunity for doctoral student research is the dissertation, although not all programs included credit allocation in their curricula for this activity. Only 10 (23%) of the programs identified dissertation seminar as part of the required program of study, and the range of credits for this curricular element was large (6 to 27), perhaps depending on the efficiency with which students could complete their projects. Materials reviewed for this project did not reveal the extent to which informal not-for-credit opportunities exist to develop research skills. It is likely, however, that there is high potential for intermittent, unstructured learning to occur in a research intensive environment.

DISCUSSION

The extent to which doctoral curricula in nursing appear to comply with the AACN recommendations regarding curricular elements that suggest programs of quality are summarized in Table 10-1. Programs evaluated in this study succeed in emphasizing development of research skills, although emphasis was clearly on quantitative methodology. The heavy focus on quantitative research reflects the current standards of mainstream doctoral education in other disciplines as well, although some might argue this unilateral approach may not always best serve the research interests of the discipline.

Student research opportunities appear to be formalized in most doctoral programs; they are an extension of the heavy emphasis on research and research skills that are a feature of doctoral education. In many ways the "hands-on"

Table 10-1
Doctoral Programs that Meet Specific AACN Criteria
for Quality*

Criteria	Percentage of Programs	(n)
Research designs, methods and techniques of analysis	100%	(44)
Theory construction	100%	(44)
History and philosophy and their relation to the development of nursing knowledge	95%	(42)
Student research opportunities	67%	(28)
Social, ethical, and political issues of importance to the discipline	59%	(26)
Data management, tools, and technology	45%	(20)
Existing substantive nursing knowledge	41%	(18)

*These percentages were gathered from the number of programs that explicitly identified course work or student experiences that demonstrated attention to the criteria noted above. The number of schools that may provide for some of these particular learning experiences, not described in their materials, may be underrepresented.

experience that students acquire during doctoral study provides the most realistic view of the research effort, and doctoral students with such exposure are more likely to become sensitive to the demands of science and the material and political realities of research.

The focus of doctoral nursing programs on research and scholarship suggests an emphasis on theory, theory testing, and theory construction. Although all programs incorporated courses or course content in nursing theory or nursing science, the number of credits tended to be small, and the particular emphasis on "theory construction" (theory analysis, theory evaluation, or theory development/construction) was unclear. Significant attention to knowledge and skills in "theory construction" may have been further incorporated into required research courses although this could not be determined from the available materials.

The inclusion of "history and philosophy and their relationship to the development of nursing knowledge" as an indicator of quality for a doctoral program may be interpreted as concern for students to have exposure to the theoretical underpinnings of science and the evolution of scientific thought. Since, in most schools (66%), the philosophy course was offered by the nursing department, one might assume that such exposure is expected within the structure of the identifiable philosophy course.

Most programs (59%) provided content in the area of social, ethical, and political issues of concern to the discipline. In programs where clinical emphasis is strong, attention to such issues was more evident; however, most doctoral students appear to have exposure to these issues.

Using AACN criteria, curricula evaluated in this study varied in the amount of emphasis placed on course content that addressed existing substantive nursing knowledge. "Existing substantive nursing knowledge," when defined as clinical nursing course content and learning experiences, is provided in fewer than half of current doctoral programs. Perhaps it is assumed that relevant clinical knowledge is obtained at the master's degree level, and that doctoral programs should focus exclusively on development and refinement of research skills. However, some master's degree programs emphasize role development and do not provide substantial expansion of existing nursing knowledge as defined in this study. Students from master's programs where advanced clinical knowledge is de-emphasized, or who have long been removed from clinical nursing, may reasonably require advanced clinical study in nursing at the doctoral level to enhance their potential to contribute to the advancement of nursing science.

Emphasis on the development or enhancement of skills in data management, tools, and technology varied widely across doctoral programs evaluated in this study. In most programs, formalized course work was not available, and exposure to these issues appears to occur in less structured learning environments. Because of the increasing complexity of technology, skill development at the level expected by those who hold the doctorate may be unlikely to occur without formalized instruction. Furthermore, while employers understand limited computer capability among long-term employees, they have reason to expect that newly hired nurses with doctoral degrees would have technologic proficiency adequate to move research agendas forward, enhance productivity, and be prepared to pass this knowledge along to their less informed colleagues or students.

Currently, instruction in data management, tools, and technology in doctoral programs in nursing may be inadequate. Improvement in this area may require substantial investment, since faculty teaching in doctoral programs may themselves rely on specialists to provide computer and technologic support to achieve their goals.

CONCLUSIONS

Each doctoral program possesses unique features that reflect the special characteristics of the faculty, the environment, and the students of its respective institution. This study focused more narrowly on the formalized structure of programs of study available in printed literature which does not fully capture the richness of doctoral education. While most doctoral programs in this country appear to possess curricular elements of quality previously identified by AACN with respect to curricular issues in the areas of research, theory construction, and philosophy, there was much more variation in the curricular content focusing on areas of substantive nursing knowledge, and data management, tools, and technology.

REFERENCES

American Association of Colleges of Nursing. (1987). Indicators of quality in doctoral programs in nursing. *Journal of Professional Nursing, 3*, 72–74.

Downs, F.S. (1989). Differences between the professional doctorate and the academic/ research doctorate. *Journal of Professional Nursing, 5*, 261–265.

Grace, H.K. (1989). Issues in doctoral education in nursing. *Journal of Professional Nursing, 5*, 266–270.

Loomis M. (1985). Emerging content in nursing: An analysis of dissertation abstracts and titles. *Nursing Research, 34,* 113–118.

Meleis, A. (1988). Doctoral education in nursing: Its present and its future. *Journal of Professional Nursing, 4,* 436–446.

Murphy, J.F. (1981). Doctoral education in, of, and for nursing: An historical analysis. *Nursing Outlook, 29,* 645–649.

National League for Nursing. (1988). *Graduate education in nursing.* New York: Author.

Sigma Theta Tau. (1991). Nursing doctoral programs in the United States. *Reflections,* 17, 23.

Ziemer, M., Brown, J., Fitzpatrick, M.L., Manfredi, C., O'Leary, J., Valiga, T. (in press). Doctoral programs in nursing: Their philosophy and curricula. *Journal of Professional Nursing.*